THE
FREQUENT FIBER COOKBOOK

Easy and Delicious **Recipes** and **Tips** for People on a High Fiber Diet

Norene Gilletz
Author of *Norene's Healthy Kitchen* and *Healthy Helpings*

Mandy Erickson
Food Reviewer, *San Francisco Chronicle*

YOUR HEALTH PRESS | Second Edition

The Frequent Fiber Diet Cookbook: Delicious Recipes and Tips for People on a High Fiber Diet
Your Health Press

Important Notice:
The purpose of this book is to educate. It is sold with the understanding that the author and publisher shall have neither liability nor responsibility for any injury caused or alleged to be caused directly or indirectly by the information contained in this book. While every effort has been made to ensure its accuracy, the book's contents should not be construed as medical advice. Each person's health needs are unique. To obtain recommendations appropriate to your particular situation, please consult a qualified healthcare provider.

Design of print and digital editions: Anita Janik-Jones
Cover photo: istockphoto.com

ISBN: 978-0-9851568-7-9

OTHER BOOKS BY NORENE GILLETZ

The New Food Processor Bible: 30th Anniversary Edition, Whitecap (2011)

Norene's Healthy Kitchen, Whitecap (2007)

The PCOS Diet Cookbook, Delicious Recipes and Tips for Women with PCOS on the Low GI Diet, Your Health Press (2007)

Healthy Helpings, Whitecap (2006)

The Low Iodine Diet Cookbook, Easy and Delicious Recipes and Tips for Thyroid Cancer Patients, Your Health Press (2005)

MicroWays, Gourmania (1989)

Second Helpings, Please!, Montreal Jewish Women International (1968)

TABLE OF CONTENTS

PART 2: COOKING AND RECIPES

WHAT IS A "HIGH FIBER" DIET?

You're hearing about high fiber diets everywhere you turn, from health magazines to commercials for bran cereal. Perhaps your doctor has advised that you start eating a high fiber diet.

But what does that mean? How much fiber makes a diet high in fiber, and how do you fit it all into the day? How does a high fiber diet affect your health?

This book answers these questions and many more. You'll learn the benefits of a diet high in fiber, the amount of fiber you need, tips for increasing fiber in the diet, shopping for high fiber cooking, ordering high fiber meals in a restaurant, and feeding children fiber-rich foods. Most important, you'll find over 350 delicious, easy-to-prepare high fiber recipes and variations—familiar favorites as well as exciting new dishes.

Increasing the fiber in your diet will start you on a tasty adventure of expanding your cooking skills and experimenting with new recipes and ingredients. It may seem daunting, but take heart: A higher-fiber diet—and better health—is easier than you think.

BENEFITS OF A HIGH FIBER DIET

Eating a diet high in fiber improves your health in a number of ways. Fiber helps lower LDL or "bad" cholesterol in your blood. Fiber also bulks up your stool, preventing constipation and lowering the risk of hemorrhoids and gastro-intestinal diseases. A diet rich in fiber helps keep blood sugar levels low and may reduce your risk of developing diabetes—or help you control your diabetes if you have it; it also lowers the glycemic index of food. Fiber helps you feel full longer, causing you to eat less and lose weight. A high fiber diet may prevent certain types of cancer. And a diet full of fiber, because it includes plenty of fruits, vegetables, and whole grains, is one filled with healthful nutrients such as vitamins, antioxidants, and minerals.

Researchers are constantly finding more benefits to a high fiber diet, but it's now clear that eating plenty of fiber extends life and improves health. Regardless of your age or physical condition, eating a high fiber diet is a smart idea.

WHAT IS FIBER?

Fiber is a catch-all term for a class of carbohydrates that exist in all plants. These carbohydrates form the rigid material that gives plants their shape: They keep asparagus standing upright and divide citrus fruit into sections. Although fiber is a carbohydrate, it is indigestible—the body passes it through the digestive system unchanged. Because it is indigestible, fiber contains no calories.

Fiber generally falls into two categories: soluble and insoluble. Soluble fiber is so-called because it dissolves in water, becoming gelatinous. Soluble fiber is found in oats (it gives cooked oatmeal its characteristic gumminess), apples (in the form of pectin, which is used to make jelly thick), and most other fruits, vegetables, and grains. Soluble fiber binds to fatty substances, carrying them through the digestive system and out of the body as waste. For this reason, soluble fiber appears to help lower blood cholesterol levels. It also helps regulate blood sugar, because it traps carbohydrates and slows their absorption and digestion.

Insoluble fibers give plants their chewy texture: the coating on brown rice, for example, or the outer peel of a broccoli stalk. These fibers do not dissolve in water, though they hold onto it, like a sponge. This quality causes insoluble fibers to bulk up stools as well as soften them, moving waste quickly through the digestive track. When waste passes rapidly through the digestive system, potentially harmful substances spend less time in the intestines, possibly reducing the risk of cancer and other diseases. Also, when stools are soft, they pass from the body easily and regularly, preventing constipation. And they require less straining to eliminate, so painful hemorrhoids aren't as likely to form.

Whatever your reasons for starting a high fiber diet, don't worry too much about soluble versus insoluble fiber because both are important for health. And most high fiber foods contain both types of fiber: The skin of an apple is insoluble, while much of its interior is soluble. And oats, though loaded with soluble fibers, include the tough outer membrane of the grain, an insoluble fiber.

Fiber is not found in animal sources, such as meat, eggs or dairy products, or in oils. Fiber is found only in plants. Some of the best sources are legumes such as beans, lentils and peas; whole grains such as whole-wheat and brown rice; vegetables such as broccoli, peas, corn and carrots; and fruit such as pears, apples, figs and berries. This is a short list, however: Most plant sources, as long as grains are kept whole, are good sources of fiber.

Fiber supplements are generally a poor way to increase the amount of fiber in your diet. These supplements often do not supply enough fiber. And much of the benefit of a high fiber diet comes from the nutrients a varied diet contains—the vitamins, minerals and antioxidants (as well as any substances scientists have yet to discover) prevalent in plant-based foods. Because it fills you up, a high fiber diet is often lower in fat and calories—a benefit you can't get from fiber supplements.

HOW MUCH FIBER IS NEEDED?

The Institute of Medicine recommends that everyone consume 14 grams of fiber for every 1,000 calories they eat. So an average diet of 2,000 calories calls for 28 grams of fiber daily. Because an adequate diet calls for 28 grams, a high fiber diet requires even more—about 35 grams. A very high fiber diet calls for an average of 50 grams a day.

You can use a range of between 35 and 50 as a rough guideline and adjust it based on your size and activity level. A college football player, for example, is possibly looking at 60 grams a day for a high fiber diet, whereas a less-active middle-age woman may require only 25 grams.

For children, the Institute of Medicine advises that 1- to 3-year-olds consume 19 grams of fiber a day and those ages 4 to 8 eat 25 grams a day. Older children have requirements close to those of adults—or more, especially if a teenager is involved in sports. If your child's doctor has recommended a high fiber diet, ask how many grams a day your child should consume.

As these amounts don't take into account any special dietary needs, check with your physician to be sure you're eating the right amount of fiber for you or serving the right amount to your child.

Some adults and children have particular problems with chronic constipation, and may be prescribed a high fiber diet, along with fiber supplements. By following the recipes and meal planning tips in this book, you may be able to achieve regularity without fiber supplements or laxatives, in consultation with your doctor.

Getting Enough Fiber

While it's helpful to know how many grams of fiber you should aim for, there's no reason to spend your day calculating calories and grams of fiber. A better approach is to adjust your diet to include whole grains and fruits and vegetables. If you include plenty of them, you won't need to worry about the numbers. Also, the recipes in this book are all high in fiber, so creating meals from these recipes guarantees a fiber-rich diet. Additionally, all recipes include a nutritional analysis that calculates fiber, and helps you gauge your intake.

Here are some easy ways to boost the fiber in your day:

- Buy 100% whole-wheat bread and whole-grain crackers.
- Serve brown rice instead of white rice.
- Sprinkle wheat bran over your morning cereal.
- Use whole-wheat pasta.
- Buy precut vegetables such as baby carrots and celery for snacks.
- Eat the peel on apples, peaches, or pears.
- Keep the skins on potatoes when you bake, fry, or mash them.
- Snack on popcorn.
- Substitute whole-wheat flour for at least half of the flour in recipes for breads, muffins, cakes, and cookies.
- Add canned or cooked beans to soups and salads.
- Include wheat bran, oat bran or rolled oats when you're making meatloaf or meatballs.
- Choose whole fruit over fruit juice.

EASING THE TRANSITION TO A HIGH FIBER DIET

If you've been eating a low fiber diet, you may find that starting a high fiber diet causes gas, bloating, and even diarrhea. To avoid these problems, introduce fiber to your digestive system slowly—as little as 2 to 4 grams a week. That works out to an apple, a cup of cooked oatmeal, or a quarter cup of cooked beans—about one serving of a high fiber food, or a half serving of a very high fiber food. For a week, substitute one of these servings for a low fiber food each day. On week 2, you can substitute two servings every day; week 3, three servings and so on.

Be sure to drink plenty of fluids along with your high fiber meals. Fiber absorbs water, so you'll need to add more to your diet to keep your stool soft.

If beans continue to cause problems with gas, don't give up on them. Eat them in smaller portions if you must. You can also get rid of many of the compounds that cause gas: Soak dry beans overnight, then discard the soaking water and refill the pot with water from the tap before you cook them. Be sure to cook them until they're completely soft. When you're using canned beans, drain off the liquid in the can.

Ultimately, this cookbook isn't just full of beans! It's filled with a range of recipes and tips that should get you the "frequent fiber miles" you need to stay healthy.

THE HIGH FIBER CUPBOARD: HOW TO SHOP FOR THE HIGH FIBER DIET

If you've read the Introduction, you know that certain foods will boost the fiber content of your diet. This chapter will help you shop for those foods. You'll also learn how to interpret food labels to determine whether the product you're buying is in fact high fiber.

We're going to explore this chapter like we're making our way through the supermarket, so grab a cart and let's go shopping!

LABELS

Laws limit food manufacturers on what they can say on their packages—they can't claim that something is high fiber when it contains very little fiber. But product titles and descriptions can still be confusing or misleading. The best way to know what you're eating is to look at the list of ingredients as well as the nutrition label, which shows the amount of fiber per serving.

Ingredients are listed in order of amount by weight, starting with the greatest amount and ending with the least. So a package of crackers may list flour as the first ingredient, then shortening, then salt. If the ingredient list reads "whole-wheat flour, flour, shortening, salt" you know there's more whole-wheat flour than white flour.

The nutrition information box next to the ingredients tells you how much fiber, in grams, you'll get per serving. (The fiber amount includes all types of fiber—soluble and insoluble.) Note the size of each serving, which is included at the top of the box: This amount can vary quite a bit. It could be two crackers, or it could be five crackers. To know how much fiber you'll be getting, you have to determine what is likely to be a serving for you, then do the math.

PRODUCE

Get to know this part of your supermarket well, because the produce section is where you'll find much of the goods for your new high fiber diet. Fruits and vegetables generally are great sources of fiber, though some are better than others.

Lettuce and spinach, the mainstay of salads, are made mostly of water, not fiber, so you won't be able to rely on those ingredients to boost your intake. If you like leafy green salads, pick up some vegetables such as shredded cabbage, corn, broccoli, carrots, or fruit, such as pears and apples, and add them to your salad bowl.

Precut vegetables save time in the kitchen—look for veggies ready for stir-fry; carrot sticks, bell peppers and celery ready for snacking; or precut squash for baking. Fruit often comes in its own package—it's a snack ready to eat.

When you shop for fruits and vegetables in season, you'll find them cheaper and much more flavorful. Good taste, more than anything, will win you over to a diet filled with fruits and vegetables.

CANNED FOODS

You'll also find a lot of high fiber friends in the canned food section. Canned soup can be a good source of fiber—look for chili with beans, soup made with wild rice, split pea soup, black bean soup, or any soup made with dried beans.

Canned vegetables that are good for a high fiber diet include peas, corn, sweet potatoes, and Italian pickled vegetables. Fruit and fruit cocktail are also high in fiber, though they can be loaded with sugar.

In the canned foods aisle you'll find lots of canned beans, such as pinto beans, black beans, chickpeas, and kidney beans. Stock up on these items, as canned beans are an excellent source of fiber, and you can toss them into salads and soups.

RICE, PASTA AND DRY BEANS

Choose brown rice over white rice. Some packaged rice mixes contain brown rice, also called "whole-grain rice," or wild rice (which isn't technically a rice, though it is whole grain); others have red beans and rice—all good sources of fiber.

Whole-wheat pasta is a better choice than regular pasta. You may also find pasta that's made with white flour and fortified with flax, which adds fiber.

Dry pinto beans, black beans, navy beans, lentils, chickpeas, and other legumes are excellent sources of fiber. Adding one serving of beans a day can boost your fiber intake substantially.

CEREALS

Breakfast cereals are a good way to start off the day with a load of fiber. Cereal manufacturers have developed cold cereals that are loaded with as much as 10 grams of fiber a serving. Some fiber-rich brands are Grape Nuts, Raisin Bran, All-Bran, Shredded Wheat, and Fiber One.

Hot cereals that are full of fiber include oatmeal (old-fashioned as well as instant) and mixed-grain cereals, such as five-grain, seven-grain or nine-grain (a mix of whole grains such as oats, rye, barley, and brown rice).

BREAD

Bread can be tricky. The label may say nine-grain or twelve-grain, but that doesn't mean the bread is high fiber. A nine-grain bread could be mostly white flour with a little bit of nine-grain cereal thrown in. Also, bread that's brown may be made with white flour and dyed with caramel or molasses. And the label may say "whole-wheat," but it could still contain mostly white flour. This is especially true for whole-wheat bagels.

Read the label—the ingredients list as well as the grams of fiber per slice (again, note the serving size: Some manufacturers consider one slice a serving, while others call two slices a serving).

Bakers are now producing white whole-wheat-bread. This is a grain that's white in color, so it looks like white bread, but contains all the fiber of whole-wheat. There are also white or refined-flour breads with added flax, which may be helpful if you're trying to boost the fiber in a child's diet.

BAKING INGREDIENTS

Choose whole-wheat flour over white flour. You may be able to find whole-wheat pastry flour, which is made from a type of wheat that has less protein and leads to a lighter crumb. Whole-wheat pastry flour is good for cookies, cakes, and quick breads. For breads that rise or require a bread machine, use regular whole-wheat flour.

As for baking mixes, there are some bran muffin mixes on the market. Buckwheat pancake mixes can be high in fiber, but check the label to be sure buckwheat is the first ingredient.

FATS AND OILS

No fats or oils contain fiber, but the fat or oil you choose is important if you're dealing with other health issues in connection with a high fiber diet. Heart-healthy fats include olive oil, canola oil, flax seed oil, peanut oil, soybean oil, and avocado oil—all oils that are high in monounsaturated fats. Olive oil has a strong flavor, so it's good for salad dressing and for drizzling on bread or pasta. The other oils, which have little flavor, are good for baking and sautéing.

If you're trying to cut down on calories, nonstick cooking sprays are great for coating saucepans or muffin or bread tins. They keep food from sticking but add very little fat.

BEVERAGES

Sodas and fruit juices add calories to your diet without adding fiber. Prune juice and V8 juice contain some fiber, but not as much as the prunes or vegetables would provide if you ate them whole. The best beverage to have with high fiber meals is water. Increasing water intake is important when adapting to a high fiber diet.

MEAT, FISH AND DAIRY

Animal proteins—poultry, fish, meat, eggs, milk, and cheese—contain no fiber, so a diet that leans too heavily on these ingredients will be low in that department. Choosing lower-fat meats such as skinless chicken, fish, and lean beef as well as exotic meats such as veal, bison and other lean cuts will employ fewer of your day's allotted calories and let you fit more high fiber foods into your diet. For the same reason, lower fat dairy products such as low-fat milk, cottage cheese, and ricotta are a better choice than whole milk and other cheeses.

SNACKS AND CRACKERS

Granola bars are taking up a lot of space these days on supermarket shelves. They're generally high in fiber, as they're typically made with oats, nuts, and dried fruit, but they're also high in sugar, so tread carefully. Be sure to check the fiber content on the label, as some bars that are marketed as healthful granola bars are really candy bars in disguise.

Many crackers are a good source of insoluble fiber, including Triscuits, Wasa crispbread, and whole-wheat matzo. As with granola bars, be sure to read the label, because many crackers that appear to be high fiber are in fact not. Crackers can also be loaded with fat and sugar.

Dried fruit, such as raisins, "craisins" (dried cranberries), figs, and cherries, are good sources of fiber. Freeze-dried vegetables have also made an appearance in some stores: These are peas, tomatoes, beans, carrots, and other veggies dried to a crisp. They're satisfyingly crunchy, like potato chips, but full of fiber and lacking the fat.

Fiber-wise, the best cookies you'll likely find on a supermarket shelf are Fig Newtons and oatmeal raisin. Some markets may carry more healthful brands made with whole-wheat flour.

Other high fiber snacks include popcorn and nuts, though these can also be high in fat and salt. Popcorn that you pop yourself in a hot-air popper, without any added salt or butter, is a healthful alternative.

DELI

Your supermarket's deli likely carries a three-bean salad, a fruit salad, and a veggie salad—all good choices for part of a healthful meal.

BULK FOODS

If your supermarket carries bulk foods, look for oats, whole-wheat flour, whole-wheat pastry flour, dried beans, brown rice, nuts, and dried fruit. The advantage to bulk foods is that they are usually cheaper than packaged foods. Health food stores often have unusual ingredients in the bulk foods department, such as brown rice flour, chickpea flour, oat bran, flax, black rice, red rice, quinoa, flaxseeds, and spelt. These ingredients are great substitutes for wheat and wheat flour if you have allergies or other conditions that prevent you from eating wheat. Even if you don't, you can have fun experimenting with a variety of whole grains such as bulger, kasha (buckwheat groats), whole wheat couscous, quinoa, and wheat berries.

FROZEN FOODS

The freezer case is an excellent source of fruit in the winter, when little fresh fruit is available. Berries, which are loaded with fiber, freeze well and make great smoothies, pies, and cobblers.

The same is true for vegetables: Look for corn, green beans, and peas when they're no longer in season, as well as broccoli, edamame (whole soy beans in the pod), lima beans, and vegetable mixes.

Some frozen waffles are now made with whole grains, though they don't offer as much fiber as many cereals and breads.

Frozen dinners, even the ones touted as being healthful, are usually geared toward people looking to lower the fat and calories in their diet, not those hoping to increase the fiber. As a result, the meals usually contain little fiber. You will likely find some good options in health food stores: Look for Indian curries made with beans or lentils.

One freezer selection that's high in fiber is vegetarian burgers (e.g. Boca Burgers Garden Burgers, or Dr. Praegar's Vegetarian Burgers).

Farmers Markets

Sample a tomato that you bought in a large supermarket, then head to a farmers market and taste one there. Likely you're thinking, How can they both be called a tomato?

The difference is shipping. Large supermarkets and supermarket chains purchase produce far from the market, so they pick tomatoes when they're still green and hard and won't turn to mush during the ride to the produce aisle. Farmers who sell their goods in farmers markets pick their tomatoes when they're ripe, usually the day before they sell them, and the difference in flavor is worlds apart.

If you haven't been much of a produce eater until this point, farmers markets may make a believer out of you. It's not just tomatoes: The produce at these markets is always in season, usually very fresh and often organic—three factors that lead to better quality and taste.

Another benefit is that farmers often give out samples of their produce, so you can taste your way through the market and find your favorites.

Farmers markets are sprouting up all over, in cities big and small. They often operate only during the summer and fall, though some are year-round, and are usually one day a week. Check with your local government to see where farmers markets are and when they are open.

Seasons for Fruits and Vegetables

Spring	Summer
Apricots	Beets
Asparagus	Blackberries
Lettuce	Blueberries
Peas	Corn
Pineapple	Cucumber
Spinach	Eggplant
Strawberries	Green Beans
	Nectarines
	Peaches
	Plums
	Raspberries
	Tomatoes
	Watermelon
	Zucchini

Fall	Winter
Acorn Squash	Chestnuts
Apples	Grapefruit
Butternut Squash	Leeks
Cauliflower	Oranges
Figs	Radishes
Grapes	Tangerines
Mushrooms	Turnips
Parsnips	
Pears	
Pomegranates	
Pumpkins	
Sweet Potatoes	

CHAPTER TWO

A SAMPLE HIGH FIBER MENU

The following three-day menu shows what a high fiber diet looks like in real life. This is just an example of a "frequent fiber" lifestyle. Mix and match to suit your tastes.

DAY ONE
Breakfast
High fiber cereal with milk
Fresh fruit

Mid-Morning Snack
An orange

Lunch
Luscious Lentil Soup (see page 77)
Whole-wheat crackers
Carrot Almond Salad (see page 86)

Mid-Afternoon Snack
Trail Mix (see page 355)

Dinner
Nutty-Baked Chicken (see page 252)
Oven-Roasted Asparagus (see page 216)
Company Stuffed Spuds (see page 203)

Dessert (optional)
Berry Mango Sherbet (see page 303)

DAY TWO
Breakfast
Refrigerator Bran Muffins (see page 57)
Fruit Smoothies (see page 60)

Mid-Morning Snack
Popcorn

Lunch
Penne Pesto with Tuna and Veggies (see page 150)

Mid-Afternoon Snack
Carrot and celery sticks with *Basic Skinny Dip* (see page 110)

Dinner
Black Bean, Barley and Vegetable Soup (see page 174)
Pumpernickel Rolls (see page 47)
Green salad with shredded cabbage, carrots and broccoli florets

Dessert (optional)
Poached Pears (see page 314)

DAY THREE
Breakfast
Omelet with broccoli, bell peppers and onion
Oatmeal Wheat Germ Bread (see page 45)

Mid-Morning Snack
Strawberries

Lunch
Hummus Wraps (see page 116)
Israeli Salad (see page 93)

Mid-Afternoon Snack
Anytime Breakfast Cookies (see page 28)

Dinner
Secret Ingredient Sweet and Sour Meatballs (see page 268)
Brown rice
Sesame Green Beans (see page 222)

Dessert (optional)
Banana Cake (see page 334)

CHAPTER THREE

HIGH FIBER ON THE TOWN

Your cupboard, refrigerator, and fruit bowl are brimming with high fiber staples and snacks; you're ready to whip up breakfast, make a lunch, and prepare a lavish dinner—all loaded with fiber. But what do you do when you're out with friends and family for a special meal? Or grabbing a bite with coworkers at lunchtime?

While one lower fiber meal now and then won't spell disaster, eating out on a regular basis means you'll have to fulfill some of your fiber needs at restaurants. Fortunately, most dining establishments are used to adjusting orders for special diets and allergies, so you can usually ask for vegetables instead of a green salad, or a whole-wheat bun for your burger. Don't be shy: Mix and match the menu to create a meal filled with fiber.

CHOOSING A RESTAURANT

Some restaurants are just going to be more fiber-friendly than others, so check out the menu posted in the doorway or go online (most restaurants now have their menus posted on their Web sites). Eateries that score high on the fiber meter offer vegetables other than leafy green salad, fruit, whole grains, and beans. The more options on the menu, the more likely you'll be able to build a meal filled with fiber.

Breakfast

If bran muffins are on the menu, you're golden. Buckwheat or whole-wheat pancakes are also good. Otherwise, an omelet or a scramble with lots of vegetables is a fine choice. Opt for "wheat" toast (restaurant-speak for whole-wheat toast) and a side of fruit rather than potatoes.

Lunch

Most sandwich shops offer a choice of bread that includes whole-wheat or nine-grain so, obviously, go with one of those. The lettuce and tomato on the sandwich score close to zero in fiber world, so don't count on them to boost your fiber intake. Instead, add a piece of fruit, a bag of baby carrots, or a three-bean salad.

Dinner: Appetizers

Good salad options are ones that contain more than leafy greens. A salad with pears and walnuts, or one tossed with chickpeas, kidney beans, broccoli, and shredded carrots will work well. Any salad made with vegetables or fruit is a good choice, as is a crudité platter of raw vegetables and a dip. Cæsar salad, or any tossed salad consisting mostly of lettuce and croutons, contains little fiber. Deep-fried vegetables—artichokes, especially, but also green beans or tempura vegetables—can be full of fiber, though also full of fat.

Black bean soup, split pea soup, or any other soup made with beans will be full of fiber. Vegetable soups, such as borscht, carrot or corn, are also good choices.

Dinner: Entrées

Even if the entrée you're salivating over is pure meat, you can construct a high fiber meal with side dishes like baked beans, coleslaw, and corn, or minestrone and a garden salad. Ask to substitute high fiber side dishes if the entrée doesn't include them: A baked potato, because it includes the skin, is a better option than mashed potatoes, French fries, or white rice. Carrots, broccoli, or corn are better than spinach. Good entrée options are any that include beans, whole grains, or a hefty amount of vegetables, such as chili with beans, pasta primavera or tabbouleh salad.

Dinner: Dessert

If you're hankering for sweets, go with a fruit-based dessert: apple, cherry, or berry pie; baked apple or poached pear; ice cream or frozen yogurt with a fresh fruit topping. A fruit crisp topped with oats or nuts is a great choice. Key lime or lemon meringue pie may contain fruit, but it offers very little fiber. A chocolate torte made with nuts has a small amount of fiber.

HIGH FIBER AROUND THE WORLD

Every cuisine has its advantages and challenges for those sticking with a high fiber diet. Let's take a look at some of them to see how to get the most fiber in a meal.

American

The classic burger-and-fries meal is woefully low in fiber. But you can up the intake by asking for a whole-wheat bun and sweet potato fries instead of French fries—options that are increasingly available. A garden burger, made with whole grains, is an excellent fiber-rich choice. If there's barbecue on the menu, it's likely that beans and coleslaw—both high in fiber—will be on the menu, too. Chili, as long as it includes beans, is always a good option.

American Fast Food

Fast food is almost uniformly lacking in fiber. While some places offer salads, these are usually lettuce salads that are weak in that area. Better choices are coleslaw, baked beans, and corn—if you can find them.

Chinese

Chinese food offers plenty of vegetables, which is great news for fiber consumers. But the plethora of white rice won't help your fiber intake. Some restaurants will serve brown rice—it never hurts to ask, even if it doesn't say so on the menu. Good meal choices include veggie-laden stir-fry dishes such as beef with broccoli, kung pao chicken, or mixed vegetables. Chinese chicken salad, if it's made with cabbage and other vegetables, is a good choice; if made with lettuce, it's not. Dim sum is almost entirely lacking in fiber.

French

The French don't care much for whole grains, so you won't find your fiber there. But they do love lentils and other beans—a great source of fiber—along with vegetables and salads. A simple lettuce salad won't offer much in the way of fiber, but salad Niçoise, with green beans and tomatoes, is a fine choice. Ratatouille, made of zucchini, eggplant, tomatoes, bell peppers, and onions, is a delicious stew that's almost nothing but fiber. Cassoulet, a classic dish of meats and white beans, is also excellent, both fiber- and taste-wise. For dessert, tart tatin, made with apples, is fiber-rich, as are any baked goods containing berries or cherries.

Greek

Ask if the restaurant carries whole-wheat pita; if so, you're in good stead. For starters, go with a Greek salad, hummus, or a dish with fava or other beans. Dolmas (graped leaves stuffed with rice) and spanakopita (spinach and feta cheese baked in phyllo) are also good choices. Greek cooks are fond of artichokes and eggplant, which are a good source of fiber, so take advantage if you find them on the menu. Stuffed peppers and zucchini are also good sources.

Indian

You're in fiber heaven here—even the bread can be fiber rich. Chapatis, made with whole-wheat flour, and papadum, made of lentils, are great sources of fiber. Opt for these breads over white rice or white-flour naan. The many vegetable and bean stews of Indian cooking provide plenty of fiber options. Choose the mixed vegetable or okra curries, and any dal, or bean, dish. Saag paneer, spinach with cheese squares, is a popular, but fiber-poor option. For dessert, you may encounter carrot halva—a delicious pudding made of shredded carrots that's fiber rich.

Italian

Italian cuisine is generally not a fiber-hunter's find. But there are a few good choices: Start with an antipasto platter if it includes beans and pickled vegetables such as artichokes, green beans, or cauliflower. Choose minestrone soup, which nearly always contains beans. Vegetable salads are sometimes available, as are pasta primavera, vegetarian lasagna, and eggplant parmesan. Opt for vegetables as a side dish rather than a lettuce salad. If you're dining in a pizza joint, likely the best you can do is throw all the veggies you can—broccoli, peppers, onions, tomatoes, artichoke hearts—on your pie. A few pizzerias have a whole-wheat crust option, so go for it if you find it.

Japanese

Japanese restaurants in the West are often poor in fiber, given their emphasis on fish and white rice. Sushi may be great for the heart and the waistline, but it's lacking in the fiber department. Most Japanese places still offer some fiber, however, in the form of tempura vegetables, seaweed salad, and the newly popular edamame—soybeans boiled in the shell. You may also find soba noodles, which are made with whole-grain buckwheat flour. Brown-rice sushi bars do exist, so if you find one, dig in!

Mexican

Because of its dependence on pinto and black beans, Mexican food can be a great source of fiber. Almost every entrée comes with a side of beans, so that's wonderful news (the lettuce salad that often accompanies Mexican meals contains a negligible amount). Burritos, because they contain beans, are usually better for fiber consumption than tacos. However, fish tacos often include curtido, or cabbage salad, so they can be a fine choice. Salsas made of raw chopped vegetables will add some fiber, as will guacamole. Nachos, if they include beans and salsa, are also good.

Middle Eastern

Many popular Middle Eastern dishes are loaded with fiber. The classic appetizer platter of hummus (chickpea dip), baba ganoush (eggplant dip), tabbouleh (whole-grain cracked wheat salad), falafel (ground beans formed into balls and fried), and dolmas will serve up plenty of fiber. Vegetable kebabs are also good sources. Baklava, with its nut filling, adds a little fiber.

Thai and Vietnamese

Food from this corner of the world is loaded with vegetables, so take advantage of them. Spring rolls, salads made of green papaya, and stir-fry dishes or curries that contain plenty of veggies are all good choices. Pho, the popular beef and rice-noodle soup, is very low in fiber.

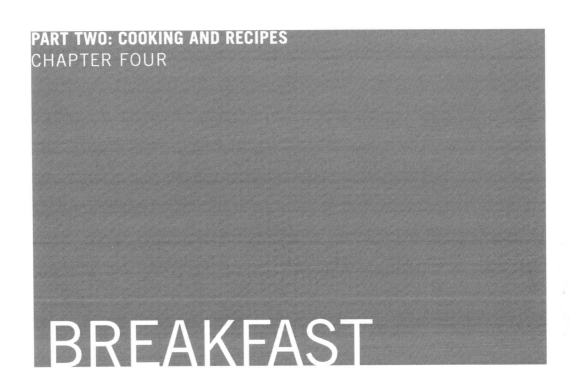

PART TWO: COOKING AND RECIPES
CHAPTER FOUR

BREAKFAST

WHAT'S INSIDE

■ CEREALS

Thanks to the many bran-based breakfast cereals available, it's easy to start the day with a load of fiber. Cold cereals that'll do the trick include Shredded Wheat, All-Bran, Bran Buds, 100% Bran, and Fiber One, as well as granola (see the recipe on page 29). If you throw in berries, kiwis, peaches, or sliced bananas, you'll add even more fiber along with vitamins and antioxidants.

Hot cereals such as oatmeal, oat bran, kasha, and seven-grain cereal are also fiber-rich. Those of you who aren't up to cooking in the morning will be glad to know that instant oatmeal contains about as much fiber as "old-fashioned" versions.

Anytime Breakfast Cookies

Thanks to my friend Anne Perrelli for sharing her recipe for scrumptious snacking cookies. They're great for kids of all ages and make a healthy breakfast or snack. For that just-baked taste, reheat them briefly in the toaster oven before serving.

> 2 cups coarsely crushed Bran Flakes
> 2 cups rolled oats (preferably large flake)
> 2 tbsp ground flaxseed or wheat germ
> 1 tbsp ground cinnamon
> 1 cup unsweetened applesauce
> ½ cup nonfat plain yogurt (or substitute your favorite flavor)
> 1 tsp pure vanilla extract
> ⅓ cup honey or maple syrup
> 1 large egg
> ½ cup skim milk powder
> 1 tsp baking powder
> 1 tsp baking soda
> ¼ cup dried cranberries or raisins

⅓ cup coarsely chopped dried apricots

½ cup chopped walnuts, almonds, or pecans

¼ cup sunflower seeds

1. Preheat the oven to 350°F. Line two large baking sheets with parchment paper.
2. In a medium-sized bowl, combine the Bran Flakes, oats, flaxseed, and cinnamon; set aside.
3. In a large mixing bowl, combine the applesauce, yogurt, vanilla, honey, egg, and skim milk powder; mix well. Add the baking powder and baking soda; mix until combined. Gradually add the reserved bran flake mixture to the applesauce mixture. Add the dried fruit, nuts, and sunflower seeds; mix well. Drop by rounded teaspoonfuls onto the prepared baking sheets.
4. Bake for 15 minutes or until golden.

Yield: About 5-½ dozen cookies. Freezes well for up to 4 months; reheats well.

38 calories per cookie, 6.0 g carbohydrate, 0.8 g fiber, 1 g protein, 1.2 g fat (0.1 g saturated), 3 mg cholesterol, 41 mg sodium, 51 mg potassium, 1 mg iron, 20 mg calcium

Granola

With the addition of milk or yogurt and a topping of fresh berries, this makes a tasty breakfast cereal for kids of all ages and is healthier than commercial granola. If you eat it plain, it also makes a super snack.

3 tbsp vegetable oil

½ cup honey

3 cups rolled oats

½ cup chopped almonds

½ cup chopped walnuts or pecans

½ cup coconut (preferably unsweetened)

1 tsp ground cinnamon

½ cup raisins or dried cranberries

½ cup chocolate chips

1. Preheat the oven to 350°F. Line a large baking sheet with parchment paper.
2. In a large bowl, combine the oil and honey. Add the oatmeal, almonds, walnuts, coconut, and cinnamon; mix well. Spread the mixture out on the prepared baking sheet.
3. Bake, uncovered, for 30 minutes or until toasted, stirring every 10 minutes. Watch carefully for the last few minutes to prevent burning.
4. Remove from the oven and transfer the hot mixture to a large bowl. Cool completely, stirring with a fork occasionally to break up any clumps. Stir in the raisins and chocolate chips.

Yield: About 6 cups (12 servings of ½ cup). Store in an airtight container, in a cool, dry place, for up to 2 to 3 weeks. Freezes well for up to 3 months.

247 calories per serving, 31.8 g carbohydrate, 3.5 g fiber, 4 g protein, 13.7 g fat (3.8 g saturated), 0 mg cholesterol, 4 mg sodium, 191 mg potassium, 1 mg iron, 30 mg calcium

Homemade Cereal Bars

These make a great snack for adults and kids alike. They're packed with dried fruit, cereal, and nuts or seeds, as well as chocolate chips for a special taste treat.

3 tbsp soft tub margarine
40 large marshmallows
4-½ cups toasted oat cereal (such as Cheerios or Bran Flakes)
¾ cup dried cranberries or raisins (or a combination)
¾ cup chopped dried apricots
½ cup toasted sliced almonds, peanuts, sunflower, or pumpkin seeds
½ to ¾ cup semi-sweet chocolate chips

1. In a large saucepan, melt the margarine and marshmallows together over low heat. Stir until the marshmallows are melted; remove from heat and cool slightly. (Or microwave in a large glass microwaveable bowl on high for 2 to 3 minutes, stirring every minute, until melted.)

2. Add the cereal, dried fruit, and almonds to the cooled marshmallow mixture; mix well to combine. Quickly stir in the chocolate chips.

3. Spoon the mixture into a sprayed 9- by 13-inch glass baking dish. Dampen your hands and press the mixture evenly into the pan. Chill in the refrigerator for ½ hour or until set. Cut into bars with a sharp knife. If you wait too long, they will be difficult to slice. Store in a covered container at room temperature.

Yield: 24 bars. These cereal bars freeze well for up to 3 months, but be sure to slice them before freezing.

122 calories per serving, 22.2 g carbohydrate, 1.6 g fiber, 2 g protein, 3.9 g fat (1.0 g saturated), 0 mg cholesterol, 70 mg sodium, 116 mg potassium, 2 mg iron, 32 mg calcium

Chef's Secrets

- *A Cut above the Rest:* Apricots are a good source of beta carotene and add lovely color to this recipe. The easiest way to cut up dried apricots is with kitchen scissors.
- *Nuts to You!* Did you know that a cup of almonds contains the same amount of calcium as a cup of milk? Almonds and sunflower seeds are also excellent sources of vitamin E.
- *The Seedy Truth:* Pumpkin seeds, with their sweet, nutty flavor, are available shelled and toasted, making them a quick, convenient, and healthy snack. They are a very good source of zinc and magnesium. You can add pumpkin seeds to baked goods, stir-fries, salads, and grains. To maintain their freshness, store pumpkin seeds in an airtight container in the refrigerator or freezer. They'll keep for several months.

■ PANCAKES AND PANCAKE TOPPINGS

Substitute whole-wheat flour for white flour in your favorite pancake and waffle recipes, or try one of the recipes enhanced with fruit, below. If you like to use a mix, go for one that contains most or all buckwheat flour. Applesauce is a great fiber-friendly topping for pancakes, as are the following mixed-fruit toppings.

Apple Blue-Peary Sauce

This fiber-packed dessert can be enjoyed hot or cold, chunky or smooth. It also makes a terrific topping for frozen yogurt, ice cream, or pancakes.

> 4 large apples, peeled, cored, and cut in chunks
> 2 cups blueberries (frozen or fresh)
> 2 pears, peeled, cored, and cut in chunks
> ⅓ cup water
> 3 tbsp brown sugar or granular Splenda
> 1 tsp ground cinnamon
> 1 tsp lemon juice (preferably fresh)

1. Combine all the ingredients in a large microwavable bowl. Cover and microwave on high for 6 to 8 minutes or until the fruit is tender, stirring once or twice during cooking.
2. Mash with a potato masher for a smoother consistency, or don't mash and leave it chunky. Serve hot or cold.

Yield: 6 to 8 servings. Keeps for up to a week to 10 days in the refrigerator. Freezes well for up to 3 months.

150 calories per serving, 39.1 g carbohydrate, 6.7 g fiber, 1 g protein, 0.6 g fat (0.1 g saturated), 0 mg cholesterol, 4 mg sodium, 264 mg potassium, 1 mg iron, 26 mg calcium. Sweet Choice—If you use granular Splenda instead of brown sugar, one serving contains 136 calories, 35.5 g carbohydrate, and 6.7 g fiber

Blueberry Cornmeal Pancakes

These pancakes are light and luscious. If you're using frozen blueberries, there's no need to defrost them: just stir the frozen blueberries into the batter and cook. Berry smart!

½ cup whole-wheat flour
¾ cup cornmeal
2 tbsp granulated sugar or granular Splenda
1 tsp baking powder
½ tsp baking soda
⅛ tsp salt
1 cup buttermilk (or 1 tbsp lemon juice plus enough skim milk to make 1 cup)
2 tbsp canola oil
2 large eggs (or 6 tbsp liquid egg whites)
1 cup blueberries (fresh or frozen)

1. Combine the flour, cornmeal, sugar, baking powder, baking soda, and salt in a large mixing bowl or food processor fitted with the steel blade; mix well. Add the buttermilk, oil, and eggs. Whisk together, or process for 8 to 10 seconds, until just smooth and blended. Gently stir in the blueberries with a rubber spatula.
2. Spray a large nonstick skillet or griddle with cooking spray. Heat over medium heat for 2 minutes or until a drop of water skips on its surface.
3. Drop the batter, using a scant ¼ cup for each pancake, into the skillet. Cook on medium heat for 2 to 3 minutes, until bubbles appear on top. Turn the pancakes over with a spatula and lightly brown the other side for 2 to 3 minutes. Transfer to a plate and keep warm. Repeat with the remaining batter, spraying the skillet between batches.

Yield: About 20 three-inch pancakes. Keeps for 2 days in the refrigerator; reheats well. Freezes well for up to 2 months. Delicious topped with additional berries, yogurt, or maple syrup (regular or light).

63 calories per pancake, 9.2 g carbohydrate, 0.9 g fiber, 2 g protein, 2.2 g fat (0.4 g saturated), 22 mg cholesterol, 91 mg sodium, 33 mg potassium, 0 mg iron, 30 mg calcium

Variations

- Omit the blueberries and instead add ½ cup dried cranberries or dried blueberries to the batter.
- **Dairy-Free Pancakes:** Instead of buttermilk, use orange juice. Or combine 1 tbsp lemon juice with enough soymilk to equal 1 cup.
- **Alphabet Pancakes:** Children love when you write their initials with pancake batter. Put the batter into a re-sealable plastic bag and cut an opening in the bottom corner. Carefully drizzle the batter into the hot skillet to form the desired letters of the alphabet. It's as easy as abc!
- **Happy Face Pancakes:** Kids love to make "happy faces" on their pancakes using chocolate chips for the eyes, a cherry for the nose, and dried cranberries for the smile.

Chef's Secrets

- *Batter Up!* Substitute 2 tbsp soy flour or protein whey powder for part of the flour in the batter to boost the protein content. You can also add 2 tbsp wheat germ or ground flaxseed to boost the fiber count.
- *Ready or Not?* To test if a skillet or griddle is hot enough, sprinkle with a few drops of water. If the water sizzles and bounces off, your pan is hot enough. If it evaporates, your pan is too hot.
- *Hot Stuff!* Place cooked pancakes in a 250°F oven to keep warm. Or reheat pancakes in the microwave, allowing 15 seconds per pancake on high.
- *Frozen Assets:* Microwave frozen pancakes on high for 20 to 25 seconds per pancake, until hot. (There's no need to thaw first!)

Cinnamon Apple Pancakes

These dairy-free pancakes are truly delicious. Make extra and freeze them—they'll reheat in seconds in the microwave. Check out the Variations on page 36.

⅔ cup whole-wheat flour

⅔ cup all-purpose flour

2 tbsp granular sugar or granular Splenda

1 tsp ground cinnamon

¼ tsp salt

1 tsp baking powder

½ tsp baking soda

1-¼ cups unsweetened apple juice

2 tbsp canola oil

2 egg whites (or 1 large egg)

2 apples, peeled, cored, and grated

1. Combine the flours, sugar, cinnamon, salt, baking powder, and baking soda in a large mixing bowl or food processor fitted with the steel blade; mix well. Add the juice, oil, and egg whites. Whisk together, or process for 8 to 10 seconds, just until smooth and blended. Don't overmix. Gently stir in the grated apples with a rubber spatula.

2. Spray a large nonstick skillet or griddle with cooking spray. Heat over medium heat for 2 minutes or until a drop of water skips on its surface.

3. Drop the batter, using a scant ¼ cup for each pancake, into the skillet. Cook the pancakes on medium heat for 2 to 3 minutes or until bubbles appear on top. Turn the pancakes over with a spatula and lightly brown the other side for 2 to 3 minutes. Transfer to a plate and keep warm. Repeat with the remaining batter, spraying the skillet between batches. Serve warm.

Yield: About 20 three-inch pancakes. Keeps for 2 days in the refrigerator; reheats well. Freezes well for up to 2 months.

63 calories per pancake, 11.2 g carbohydrate, 1 g fiber, 1 g protein, 1.6 g fat (0.1 g saturated), 0 mg cholesterol, 91 mg sodium, 60 mg potassium, 0 mg iron, 19 mg calcium

Variations

- *Top It Up:* Top pancakes with yogurt and homemade chunky applesauce.
- *Multiply Your Options:* Fresh or frozen blueberries, blackberries, or strawberries add flavor and fiber to pancakes. If berries are frozen, you don't need to thaw them first. Instead of apples, add 1-½ cups berries to batter. Or add chopped pears, peaches, or nectarines for a twist.
- *Pom Power:* Use pomegranate juice instead of apple juice.
- *Go for Protein:* To add a protein boost to the pancake batter, add 1 to 2 tbsp protein whey powder and reduce the amount of flour accordingly.
- *Soy Good:* To increase your intake of soy, use soymilk instead of apple juice.
- *Dairy Good:* Combine equal parts of nonfat yogurt and skim milk, and mix well. Use instead of apple juice.
- *Lighten Up!* For light, fluffy pancakes, substitute club soda for up to half of the liquid.

Homemade Fruit Pancakes

This simple recipe is quick to mix up for a quick breakfast or light lunch.

1-¾ cups whole-wheat flour
1 tsp baking powder
½ tsp baking soda
2 egg whites (or 1 egg)
¾ cup skim milk
1 cup nonfat yogurt
2 tbsp honey or maple syrup
1 tbsp canola oil
1 cup blueberries, cranberries, or grated apple

1. Combine all ingredients except fruit in a bowl or processor and blend until smooth. Stir in fruit. Spray a large nonstick skillet with nonstick spray. Heat over medium-high heat for 2 minutes, or until a drop of water skips on its surface. Drop the batter by rounded spoonfuls onto the hot pan. Cook pancakes about 2 to 3 minutes on each side, or until brown. Repeat with remaining batter. Serve plain or top with warm maple syrup, applesauce, or a dollop of yogurt with fresh berries.

Yield: 16 to 18 pancakes. Refrigerate leftovers. These can be reheated briefly in the microwave.

85 calories per pancake, 1.1 g fat (0.1 g saturated), <1 mg cholesterol, 3 g protein, 16 g carbohydrate, 86 mg sodium, 96 mg potassium, <1 mg iron, <1 g fiber, 48 mg calcium

Mixed Fruit Compote

This delicious compote is perfect for people with diabetes. It's also a terrific topping for pancakes or a scrumptious sauce over frozen yogurt or ice cream. If you're short of one fruit, just use more of another one.

2 cups blueberries or blackberries
2 cups strawberries, hulled and halved
3 plums, pitted and sliced
3 nectarines or peaches, pitted and sliced
3 large apples (try Cortland, Spartan, or Gala), peeled, cored, and cut in chunks
1-½ cups water
½ cup granular Splenda (or to taste)
1 tsp ground cinnamon

1. Combine the berries, plums, nectarines, and apples in a large pot. You should have 8 to 9 cups of fruit. Add the water and bring to a boil. Reduce heat and simmer, partially covered, for about 20 to 25 minutes or until tender, stirring occasionally.

2.　Remove from the heat and stir in the Splenda and cinnamon. When cool, transfer to glass jars or freezer containers. Cover and refrigerate. Serve chilled.

Yield: About 8 cups (16 servings of ½ cup each). Keeps for up to 10 days in the refrigerator; reheats well. Freezes well for up to 4 months.

58 calories per serving, 14.7 g carbohydrate, 2.5 g fiber, 1 g protein, 0.3 g fat (0 g saturated), 0 mg cholesterol, 1 mg sodium, 160 mg potassium, 0 mg iron, 11 mg calcium. Sweet Choice—if made with sugar instead of Splenda, one serving contains 79 calories and 20.2 g carbohydrate.

Variations

- Raspberries, cranberries, and/or peeled peaches or pears can be substituted for any of the fruits. Frozen mixed berries are also delicious in this compote.

■ BAKED BREAKFAST DISHES

These do-ahead dishes are great for a crowd or lazy weekend mornings.

Crustless Zucchini Quiche

This treasured family recipe comes with "hugs and quiches" from Shani Bitan of Hong Kong. Her late grandmother, Ray Goldin, made this quiche for her family and now her two granddaughters make it for their children in Hong Kong and Lyon, France. Ray's recipe called for ½ cup oil, but I used half oil and half yogurt. I also used a combination of egg whites and eggs to lower the fat.

　　3 or 4 medium zucchini, cut in chunks (about 1-½ lb/750 g)
　　2 medium onions, cut in chunks
　　2 large eggs plus 4 egg whites (or 4 eggs)
　　½ cup canola oil
　　¾ cup whole-wheat flour
　　¾ tsp baking powder

2 cloves garlic (about 2 tsp minced)
½ tsp salt
½ tsp dried oregano
½ tsp dried basil
½ tsp dried thyme
1 cup grated low-fat mozzarella cheese

1. Preheat the oven to 375°F. Spray a 10-inch ceramic quiche dish with cooking spray.
2. In a food processor fitted with the steel blade, process the zucchini in batches; chop coarsely, using 5 or 6 quick on/off pulses. Transfer the chopped zucchini to a large bowl. Add the onions to the food processor and process with quick on/off pulses, until coarsely chopped. Transfer to the bowl and mix together with the chopped zucchini; set aside.
3. In the food processor bowl, process the eggs and egg whites with the oil for 5 seconds or until combined. Add the flour, baking powder, garlic, salt, oregano, basil, and thyme; process for 10 to 12 seconds or until blended. Add the cheese and process 10 seconds longer.
4. Return the reserved zucchini and onion to the processor bowl and process with several on/off pulses or until combined, scraping down the sides of the bowl as needed. (If you have a small food processor, add the flour mixture to the zucchini mixture and stir with a wooden spoon to combine.)
5. Pour the mixture into the prepared dish and spread evenly. Bake, uncovered, for 45 to 50 minutes or until golden brown.

Yield: 8 servings. Keeps for up to 2 to 3 days in the refrigerator; reheats well. Freezes well for up to 2 months.

191 calories per serving, 15.5 g carbohydrate, 2.9 g fiber, 9 g protein, 10.8 g fat (2.4 g saturated), 62 mg cholesterol, 502 mg sodium, 331 mg potassium, 1 mg iron, 178 mg calcium

Chef's Secrets

- *Timesaver:* Grandma Ray sliced the zucchini, but her granddaughters chop it in the processor.
- *Herbal Magic:* Grandma used dried parsley, her granddaughters like to use Herbes de Provence, but I use basil and thyme because I always have them in my kitchen.
- *Say Cheese!* Shani Bitan increases the cheese to 1-½ cups and uses a mixture of cheeses. Experiment with Swiss, cheddar, havarti, etc.

Lox and Bagel Cheese Strata

This do-ahead brunch dish is perfect fare for any special occasion. It's an excellent way to use up leftover bagels, or buy day-old bagels so that you can afford the lox. To save money, you can use lox bits and pieces. It's "dill-icious"!

> 5 to 6 whole-wheat bagels, cut in bite-sized pieces (about 8 cups)
> 8 oz (250 g) lox (smoked salmon), cut in bite-sized pieces
> 8 oz low-fat Swiss and/or havarti cheese (about 2 cups grated)
> 2 green onions, chopped
> 2 to 3 tbsp minced fresh dillweed
> 6 large eggs (or 4 eggs plus 4 egg whites)
> 1 cup light sour cream or plain yogurt
> 2 cups milk (skim or 1%)
> ½ tsp salt (optional)
> ¼ tsp freshly ground black pepper

1. Spray the bottom and sides of a 9- by 13-inch glass baking dish with cooking spray. Spread the bagel pieces evenly in the dish. Top with lox and sprinkle with the grated cheese, green onions, and dillweed.
2. In a medium bowl, combine the eggs, sour cream, milk, and seasonings; blend well (you can use a blender, whisk, or large food processor). Pour evenly over the bagel-cheese mixture. Cover and refrigerate for at least 1 hour. (If desired, you can prepare the recipe up to this point and refrigerate for 24 hours.)

3. Preheat the oven to 350°F. Bake, uncovered, for about 1 hour or until the mixture is puffed and golden. Remove from the oven and let it stand for 10 minutes for easier cutting. Serve with a large Cæsar or mixed garden salad.

Yield: 12 servings. Keeps for 2 to 3 days in the refrigerator; reheats well. Freezes well for up to 2 months.

277 calories per serving, 30.9 g carbohydrate, 2.2 g fiber, 20 g protein, 7.2 g fat (3.1 g saturated), 141 mg cholesterol, 761 mg sodium, 217 mg potassium, 2 mg iron, 308 mg calcium

Variations
- You can also make this using whole-wheat or multigrain bread, cut in 1-inch pieces.
- Instead of lox, use 2 cans (7-½ oz/213 g each) of sockeye salmon, drained and flaked. You could also use 1-½ cups of leftover cooked salmon. This can also be made with canned tuna.
- Other cheeses can be substituted; try Monterey Jack, cheddar, Jarlsberg, or a mixture. For a different twist, add ½ cup crumbled feta or goat cheese.

■ BREADS

If you like eggs in the morning, you can still down a high fiber breakfast by eating them with high fiber toast and fruit. Fill omelets with fiber-rich vegetables such as broccoli and asparagus.

There are plenty of high fiber breads available in the supermarket: Look for "100% whole-wheat" bread, "double-fiber" bread or white whole-wheat. Check the label to make sure it's as high in fiber as it claims. There should be at least 2 grams of fiber per slice.

Whole-wheat bagels are great if they are truly whole-wheat. Many so-called whole-wheat bagels contain just a pinch of whole-wheat flour, so check the fiber content. You can ratchet up the fiber by spreading the bagels with Healthier Hummus (page 114) rather than cream cheese.

High Fiber Bread

Thanks to Sharon Kravetsky of Winnipeg for sharing her recipe for this tasty, fiber-packed bread. Her bread machine has a super-rapid cycle that makes bread from start to finish in 59 minutes, so she uses water that is 110°F and increases the yeast to 2-½ tablespoons. I prefer to mix the dough in my bread machine, then shape and bake it conventionally, so I use room temperature water and less yeast.

8 to 9 oz water (at room temperature)
1 tsp salt
1 tbsp honey
1 tbsp canola oil
¼ cup rolled oats
½ cup ground 100% bran cereal, (about 1 cup whole cereal)
1-½ cups all-purpose flour
2-¼ tsp bread machine yeast

1. Place all the ingredients in the baking pan of a bread machine in the order given. Select the dough cycle. If the dough seems too sticky during the kneading cycle, add 1 to 2 tbsp additional flour. When the dough cycle is complete (it will take about 2 hours), the dough should reach to the top of the pan. If it doesn't, let the dough rise a few minutes longer in the machine.

2. Remove the dough from the machine and transfer it to a lightly floured surface. Knead for 1 to 2 minutes or until smooth and elastic. Pat out the dough into a 9- by 12-inch rectangle and then roll up into a cylinder from the longer side. Seal the ends by pressing down with the edge of your hand. Lengthen it into a long loaf by rolling it back and forth with your hands. Place seam-side down on a parchment paper-lined baking sheet, cover with a towel, and let rise for 1 to 1-½ hours or until slightly more than doubled.

3. Heat the oven to 375°F. Bake for 30 minutes. When the bread is done, it should sound hollow when tapped with your fingers.

Yield: 1 long loaf (about 18 slices). Freezes well for up to 3 months.

70 calories per slice, 13.9 g carbohydrate, 2.0 g fiber, 2 g protein, 1.1 g fat (0.1 g saturated), 0 mg cholesterol, 151 mg sodium, 74 mg potassium, 2 mg iron, 7 mg calcium

Chef's Secret

- *Bran Power!* Use a food processor or blender to grind the bran cereal to a flour-like consistency. It will yield a little more than ½ cup bran flour when ground.

Homemade Whole-Wheat Bread (Processor Method)
Wholesome and hearty.

1 tsp sugar
½ cup warm water (about 110°F)
1 pkg yeast (regular or quick-rise)
¾ cup skim milk (or lukewarm water)
1-⅓ cups all-purpose flour
1-½ cups whole-wheat flour (about)
¼ cup wheat germ, optional
1-½ tbsp sugar or honey
1 tsp salt
1 tbsp canola oil

1. Dissolve sugar in warm water. Sprinkle yeast over water and let stand 8 to 10 minutes. Stir to dissolve. Heat milk until lukewarm (about 40 seconds on HIGH in the microwave). Measure flours into processor bowl. Add wheat germ, sugar, salt, and oil. Process 10 seconds. Add dissolved yeast; process 10 seconds more. Add milk slowly through feed tube while machine is running. Process until dough gathers around the blades in a mass. Process 45 seconds longer. Dough should be slightly sticky. If machine slows down, add 3 or 4 tablespoons more flour.

2. Turn dough out onto a lightly floured surface. Knead for 2 minutes, until smooth and elastic. Shape into a ball and place in a large lightly greased bowl. Cover bowl with plastic wrap and let dough rise in a warm place until doubled, about 1-½ to 2 hours. Punch down.

3. Roll or pat dough on a lightly floured board into a 9- by 12-inch rectangle. Roll up jelly roll–style from the short side. Seal ends by pressing down with the edge of your hand. Place seam-side down in a sprayed 9- by 5-inch loaf pan or on a sprayed baking sheet. Cover with a towel and let rise until double, about 1 hour. Bake in a preheated 425°F oven for 25 to 30 minutes. Remove from pan; let cool.

Yield: 1 loaf (16 slices). Freezes well.

94 calories per slice, 1.2 g fat (0.1 saturated), trace cholesterol, 3 g protein, 18 g carbohydrate, 153 mg sodium, 85 mg potassium, 1 mg iron, 2 g fiber, 20 mg calcium

Variations

- **Whole-Wheat Rolls:** In Step 3, shape dough into 12 balls. Place on a sprayed or nonstick cookie sheet, cover and let rise until doubled. Bake at 375°F for 20 minutes, until golden.
- **Herb Bread:** In Step 1, add ½ tsp each of dried basil, dill, thyme, oregano, and/or rosemary to flour. Add remaining ingredients, mix, shape, and bake as directed.
- **Herbed Cheese Bread:** In Step 3, roll dough into a rectangle. Spread with 2 tsp olive oil, 2 cloves minced garlic, ⅓ cup grated Parmesan, and 2 tbsp minced onion. (You can add 2 tbsp minced fresh basil, ¼ cup minced sun-dried tomatoes, and/or red peppers.) Roll up and seal ends. Brush with an egg yolk mixed with 1 tbsp water. Sprinkle with sesame seeds. Place on a sprayed baking sheet, cover and let rise until double. Bake at 425°F 25 to 30 minutes.

- **Cinnamon Babka:** In Step 3, sprinkle dough with 1 cup cinnamon-sugar and ½ cup raisins. Roll up and slice in 1-inch pieces. Place in a sprayed 10-inch spring form pan, with buns barely touching. Brush with melted apricot jam. Cover and let rise until double. Bake at 375°F for 30 minutes.

Oatmeal Wheat Germ Bread

1 cup rolled oats (quick-cooking or regular)
2 cups boiling water
1 tsp sugar
½ cup lukewarm water (about 110°F)
1 pkg active dry yeast
¼ cup molasses
¼ cup maple syrup
2 tsp salt
2 tsp canola oil
3 cups all-purpose or bread flour
1-½ cups whole-wheat flour
½ cup wheat germ
1 egg white beaten with 1 tbsp cold water

1. Place oats in a large mixing bowl. Pour boiling water over oats and let stand for 20 minutes. Dissolve sugar in ½ cup lukewarm water. Add yeast and let stand for 10 minutes. Stir to dissolve. Add yeast mixture to oats along with molasses, maple syrup, salt, and oil. Slowly stir in flours and wheat germ; mix well. Transfer dough to a floured surface and knead for 3 or 4 minutes.

2. Place in a lightly greased large bowl, cover and let rise in a warm place for 1-½ hours. Punch down. Shape into 2 loaves; place in sprayed loaf pans. Cover and let rise until doubled, about 1 hour. Brush with egg white mixture. Preheat oven to 375°F. Bake for 40 to 45 minutes, until golden. When done, loaves will pull away from sides of pans. Remove from pans and cool on racks.

Yield: 2 loaves (32 slices). These freeze well.

93 calories per slice (1/16 loaf), 0.8 g fat (0.1 g saturated), 0 mg cholesterol, 3 g protein, 19 g carbohydrate, 150 mg sodium, 103 mg potassium, 1 mg iron, 2 g fiber, 13 mg calcium

Pumpernickel Loaves

Looks like bread but tastes like cake, so control yourself. Sharon Kravetsky of Winnipeg shared this yummy bread machine recipe with me. She wrote, "Even though this recipe has sugar, it has healthy flours, very little fat, and no eggs. Sounds healthy to me!"

  1-⅔ cups warm water (about 105°F)
  2 tbsp canola oil
  ¼ cup granulated sugar
  3 tbsp molasses
  2 tsp salt
  2-⅓ cups all-purpose flour
  1 cup whole-wheat flour
  ¾ cup rye flour
  3 tbsp unsweetened cocoa powder
  2 tsp instant coffee granules
  2 tbsp caraway seeds
  ⅓ cup dried onion flakes
  2 tsp bread machine yeast
  1 to 2 tbsp cornmeal (for dusting baking sheet)

1. Place all the ingredients except the cornmeal in the baking pan of a bread machine in the order given. Choose the dough cycle. If the dough seems too sticky during the kneading cycle, add 1 to 2 tbsp additional flour. When the dough cycle is complete (it will take about 2 hours), the dough should reach to the top of the pan. If it doesn't, let the dough rise a few minutes longer in the machine.

2. Remove the dough from the machine and shape it into 2 round loaves. Place the loaves a few inches apart on a parchment paper-lined baking sheet that has been sprinkled lightly with cornmeal. Cover with a towel and let rise for about 1 hour or until slightly more than doubled.

3. Heat the oven to 350°F. Bake about 35 minutes; when the loaves are done, they should sound hollow when tapped with your fingers. Remove from the baking sheet and let cool on a wire rack.

Yield: 2 loaves (about 24 slices). Freezes well for up to 3 months.

108 calories per slice, 21.1 g carbohydrate, 2.4 g fiber, 3 g protein, 1.7 g fat (0.2 g saturated), 0 mg cholesterol, 196 mg sodium, 143 mg potassium, 1 mg iron, 19 mg calcium

Variation

- **Pumpernickel Rolls:** In Step 2, shape the dough into 24 rolls. (You can also shape them into football-shaped logs, placing some fried onions in the middle of each roll.) Cover and let rise for 45 to 60 minutes. Bake at 325°F for 25 minutes.

Chef's Secrets

- *Sweet Treat:* Sharon uses ½ cup granulated sugar as her family loves sweeter bread. Everyone inhales it!
- *Timing Tip:* Add dried onions and caraway seeds when the machine beeps, which indicates when more ingredients can be added. The onions and seeds will retain more of their distinct flavor when added later.
- *Super Bowl!* Cut 1 inch off the top of the baked pumpernickel. Hollow out the inside, leaving a wall of bread about ½-inch thick around. Cut the bread you've removed into bite-sized cubes. Fill the hollowed-out bread with dip. Serve with crudités and bread cubes. You'll bowl them over!

■ MUFFINS

When you make a batch of muffins, you can always freeze the leftovers and zap them in the microwave for a quick breakfast. Boost the fiber and cut the fat in your favorite muffin recipe by substituting whole-wheat flour for half of the white flour and substituting Prune Purée (page 56) for half of the fat.

Apri-Oat Almond Muffins

"Oat cuisine" at its best! This combination of apricots and almonds make these muffins A-okay.

½ cup whole-wheat flour
½ cup all-purpose flour
1 cup rolled oats
1 tsp baking powder
½ tsp baking soda
1 large egg (or 2 egg whites)
¼ cup soft tub margarine or canola oil
½ cup lightly packed brown sugar
1 cup plain nonfat yogurt
½ tsp almond or pure vanilla extract
⅔ cup dried apricots, cut in small pieces
12 whole almonds

1. Preheat the oven to 400°F. Line the compartments of a muffin pan with paper liners (or spray with cooking spray).
2. In a food processor fitted with the steel blade, combine the flours, oats, baking powder, and baking soda; process for 5 seconds to combine. Add the egg, margarine, brown sugar, yogurt, and almond extract; process for 25 to 30 seconds or until smooth and blended. Stir in the apricots with a rubber spatula.

3.   Scoop the batter into the prepared muffin pan, filling each compartment about two-thirds full. Top each muffin with 1 almond. Bake for 20 to 25 minutes or until the tops are golden brown and spring back when lightly touched.

Yield: 12 muffins. Freezes well for up to 3 months.

160 calories per muffin, 24.8 g carbohydrate, 2.2 g fiber, 4 g protein, 5.5 g fat (0.7 g saturated), 18 mg cholesterol, 155 mg sodium, 147 mg potassium, 1 mg iron, 77 mg calcium

Chef's Secrets
- *Brown Sugar Substitute:* Use ½ cup granulated sugar plus 1 tbsp molasses.
- *No Yogurt?* Substitute 1 tbsp lemon juice plus skim or soymilk to make 1 cup.
- *Sharp Thinking!* To cut up apricots easily, use scissors.
- *Nuts to You!* Almonds are high in protein, fiber, calcium, vitamin E, and magnesium.

Apricot Prune Muffins
(See recipe, page 333)

Blueberry Corn Muffins
Berry photogenic! Are you wild about blueberries? Bite into these yummy muffins and say goodbye to the blues. Blueberries are supposed to improve your memory, so remember to add them to your shopping list!

1 cup cornmeal
1 cup whole-wheat flour
2 tsp baking powder
¾ tsp baking soda
⅛ tsp salt
½ cup plain nonfat yogurt
½ cup orange juice (preferably fresh)

¼ cup canola oil

½ cup granulated sugar

2 large eggs (or 1 large egg plus 2 egg whites)

1 tsp ground cinnamon

1 cup fresh or frozen blueberries (don't defrost if frozen)

1. Preheat the oven to 375°F. Line the compartments of a muffin pan with paper liners (or spray with cooking spray).
2. In a food processor fitted with the steel blade (or in a large bowl and using an electric mixer), combine the cornmeal, flour, baking powder, baking soda, and salt; process until well mixed. Add the yogurt, orange juice, oil, sugar, eggs, and cinnamon; process, using quick on/off pulses, just until smooth. Stir in the blueberries with a rubber spatula.
3. Scoop the batter into the prepared muffin pan, filling each compartment about three-quarters full. Bake for 20 to 25 minutes or until golden brown and the tops spring back when lightly touched. Cool slightly before removing from the pan.

Yield: 12 muffins. Freezes well for up to 3 months.

173 calories per muffin, 27.1 g carbohydrate, 3.4 g fiber, 4 g protein, 6.1 g fat (0.6 g saturated), 35 mg cholesterol, 206 mg sodium, 81 mg potassium, 1 mg iron, 73 mg calcium

Variation

- **Cranberry Orange Muffins:** Instead of blueberries, substitute with frozen cranberries or dried cranberries. Instead of cinnamon, substitute with 1 tsp grated orange zest.

Chef's Secrets

- *Frozen Assets:* Freeze fresh unwashed blueberries in a single layer on a baking tray, and then transfer to re-sealable plastic freezer bags for up to 3 months. Keep frozen blueberries on hand so you can make these muffins at a moment's notice.

- *Fresh, Frozen, or Dried?* Dried blueberries are also delicious in these muffins, so keep some on hand in your pantry. Dried blueberries are a better source of antioxidants than fresh or frozen. They're available dried in bulk food stores and can be stored in the pantry for several months. One-half cup of fresh or frozen blueberries is the equivalent of ¼ cup dried blueberries.

Bran-ana Sour Cream Muffins
(See recipe, page 336)

Bran and Date Muffins
Moist, low in fat, high in flavor, these are guaranteed to be a regular at your house! Originally, I was making these marvelous muffins with ¼ cup of oil, but discovered that they tasted even more delicious when I substituted Prune Purée (page 56) for part of the fat.

1-½ cups natural bran or All-Bran cereal
2 tbsp canola oil
¾–1 cup dates, cut-up
¾ cup raisins, rinsed and drained
½ cup hot water
2 tbsp Prune Purée (page 56) or applesauce
2 egg whites (or 1 egg)
1 cup buttermilk or sour milk
2 tbsp molasses or honey
1-¼ cups whole-wheat flour
⅓ cup sugar (brown or white)
1 tsp baking soda
½ tsp baking powder

1. Combine bran, oil, dates, and raisins in a large mixing bowl. Pour hot water over mixture; let cool slightly. Stir in purée, egg whites, buttermilk, and molasses. Add remaining ingredients and stir just enough to moisten dry ingredients. If you have time, let mixture stand for 20 to 30 minutes. (I usually do this while the oven is heating and I'm cleaning up.)
2. Preheat oven to 400°F. Line muffin pans with paper liners. Fill three quarters full with batter. Bake for 20 to 25 minutes, until nicely browned.

Yield: 1 dozen. These freeze well.

193 calories per muffin, 3.2 g fat (0.4 g saturated), <1 mg cholesterol, 5 g protein, 42 g carbohydrate, 227 mg sodium, 424 mg potassium, 2 mg iron, 5 g fiber, 67 mg calcium

Chef's Secrets

*   *Fiber Facts!* Bran is available in two forms, unprocessed and processed. Just compare: ½ cup unprocessed natural wheat bran (e.g., Quaker brand) contains 14 grams of dietary fiber, ½ cup of All-Bran contains 10 grams, but ½ cup of processed Bran Flakes has only 3 grams of fiber.
*   To cut up dates easily, dip scissors in flour first. This prevents sticking. (For variety, make one batch of muffins with raisins or dried apricots, make another batch with dates.)
*   My first choice is to use Prune Purée in these muffins. It takes just moments to make, adds fiber and flavor, and keeps perfectly in the fridge for at least 3 months. Do try it! You can substitute unsweetened applesauce if it's more convenient. Either one is excellent.
*   To make sour milk, mix 1 tbsp lemon juice or vinegar plus skim milk to equal 1 cup. For dairy-free recipes, substitute soy or rice milk plus lemon juice or vinegar.
*   An alternative to sour milk or buttermilk in muffin and cake recipes is to mix ½ cup of nonfat yogurt with ½ cup of water.
*   For even-sized muffins, scoop out batter with an ice cream scoop, or use a ½ cup dry measure.

- *Lee's Ever-Ready Muffin Mixture:* Lee Stillinger, one of my enthusiastic students, loves this recipe so much, she makes four times the original recipe and stores the batter in the refrigerator in an airtight container. (It keeps for about 3 weeks.) That way, she can have fresh muffins whenever she's in the mood. (If you're not quite as enthusiastic, just double the recipe!)

Cathy's Ever-Ready Honey Bran Muffins

Cathy Ternan, my exercise partner, special friend, and proofreader, shared this excellent do-ahead muffin recipe with me. I replaced part of the honey with molasses and used applesauce to replace part of the fat in these tender, tasty muffins. They're not too sweet and are packed with fiber and flavor.

6 cups natural bran, divided
1-¾ cups boiling water
½ cup canola oil
1-¾ cups honey
¼ cup molasses
½ cup unsweetened applesauce
4 eggs (or 2 eggs plus 4 egg whites)
4 cups buttermilk
5 cups whole-wheat flour
5 tsp baking soda
1 tsp salt
1 tbsp cinnamon
2 cups raisins, rinsed and drained

1. Place 2 cups of bran in a very large mixing bowl or storage container. Pour boiling water over bran, stir well to moisten and let mixture stand for about 5 minutes.

2. Add oil, honey, molasses, applesauce, eggs, buttermilk and remaining bran to bowl. Stir to combine. Sift in flour, baking soda and salt. Mix in cinnamon and raisins. Batter will keep for up to 6 weeks in the refrigerator. Bake as many muffins as needed.

3. Preheat oven to 375°F. Fill paper-lined muffin cups three-quarters full with batter. Bake for 20 to 25 minutes, until nicely browned.

Yield: About 4 dozen. These freeze well.

164 calories per muffin, 3.6 g fat (0.5 g saturated), 18 mg cholesterol, 4 g protein, 33 g carbohydrate, 266 mg sodium, 275 mg potassium, 2 mg iron, 4 g fiber, 45 mg calcium

Chef's Secrets
- Quaker Oats makes natural wheat bran, or you can buy it in bulk. Substitute all or part All-Bran cereal if you are short of natural bran.
- Optional at baking time: Add chopped dates, apples, chocolate chips, nuts, etc. to batter.
- **Oatmeal Bran Muffins:** Follow recipe above, but use 4 cups of wheat bran and 2 cups of oats (quick-cooking or regular). Replace the honey with 2 cups of firmly packed brown sugar.

Honey Almond Bran-ana Muffins

These luscious dairy-free muffins are not too sweet and are full of fiber and flavor. The whole-grain cereal, ground almonds, and flaxseed or wheat germ make them a great choice for a healthy breakfast or snack. Did you know that a cup of almonds contains the same amount of calcium as a cup of milk?

2 large eggs
2 tbsp canola oil
½ cup honey
1 tsp pure vanilla extract
1 cup All-Bran cereal

3 very ripe medium bananas (about 1-½ cups mashed)
2 tbsp water
1 cup whole-wheat flour
½ cup finely ground almonds (almond meal)
3 tbsp ground flaxseed or wheat germ
2 tsp baking powder
½ tsp baking soda

1. Preheat the oven to 375°F. Spray the compartments of a muffin pan with cooking spray.
2. In a food processor fitted with the steel blade (or in a large bowl and using an electric mixer), combine the eggs, oil, honey, and vanilla; process for 2 minutes or until light in color. Add the bran, bananas, and water; mix well. Add the flour, ground almonds, flaxseed, baking powder, and baking soda; process just until blended.
3. Scoop the batter into the prepared muffin pan, filling each compartment three-quarters full. Bake for 20 to 25 minutes or until the tops are golden brown and spring back when lightly touched.

Yield: 12 muffins. Freezes well for up to 3 months.

185 calories per muffin, 31.1 g carbohydrate, 4.7 g fiber, 5 g protein, 6.6 g fat (0.8 g saturated), 35 mg cholesterol, 160 mg sodium, 240 mg potassium, 2 mg iron, 89 mg calcium

Variation

*   **Honey Almond Bran-ana Loaf:** Pour batter into a sprayed 9- by 5-inch loaf pan and spread evenly. Bake at 350°F for 50 to 60 minutes. When done, a cake tester or toothpick, when inserted into the center, should come out clean.

"Nut"-rition Notes

- *Nuts about Almonds!* Just one ounce of almonds contains half the daily requirement for vitamin E. Almonds are also a good source of magnesium, dietary fiber, and plant compounds that can help control blood cholesterol. The brown skin on almonds contains flavonoids, but almonds without the skin are also a healthy choice.

Prune Purée

This is a fabulous fat substitute to use in baking! It's quick and easy to make, plus it's much cheaper than the commercial version. Prune Purée is packed with potassium and fiber.

>2 cups pitted prunes (about 36)
>1 cup hot water

1. Combine prunes and hot water in a bowl. Cover and let stand for 5 minutes, until plump. In a processor or blender, process prunes with water until smooth, about 1 minute. Scrape down sides of bowl several times.

Yield: About 2 cups. Store tightly covered in the fridge for up to 3 months, or freeze for 6 months.

20 calories per tbsp, 0 g fat (0 g saturated), 0 mg cholesterol, trace protein, 5 g carbohydrate, <1 mg sodium, 63 mg potassium, trace iron, <1 g fiber, 4 mg calcium. 304 calories per cup, 0.7 g fat (0.1 g saturated), 0 mg cholesterol, 3 g protein, 80 g carbohydrate, 8 mg sodium, 948 mg potassium, 3 mg iron, 12 g fiber, 67 mg calcium

Refrigerator Bran Muffins

If you like freshly baked healthy muffins, this fiber-packed recipe is perfect for you! Prepare the batter and bake as few or as many muffins as you like. Refrigerate the leftover batter in an airtight container for up to 3 weeks so you can enjoy fresh-from-the-oven muffins in less time than it takes to visit the bakery. Brew a big pot of tea, use one cup in the batter and pour a cup to sip while mixing up the batter. Tea-licious!

3 cups bran buds with psyllium (or natural bran, All-Bran cereal, or Bran Flakes)
⅓ cup canola oil
⅓ cup unsweetened applesauce
1 cup raisins
1 cup dried cranberries
1 cup hot tea (green tea is a great choice)
2 large eggs (or ½ cup liquid egg substitute)
2 cups buttermilk (or 2 tbsp lemon juice plus skim or soymilk to equal 2 cups)
½ cup lightly packed brown sugar
½ cup molasses or honey
2-½ cups whole-wheat or all-purpose flour
2 tsp ground cinnamon
2 tsp baking soda
1 tsp baking powder

1. Preheat the oven to 375°F. Line the compartments of muffin pan(s) with paper liners (or spray with cooking spray).
2. Combine the bran, oil, applesauce, raisins, and cranberries in a large mixing bowl. Pour the hot tea over mixture and let stand for 5 minutes. Stir in the eggs, buttermilk, brown sugar, and molasses. Add the flour, cinnamon, baking soda, and baking powder. Stir briefly, just until combined. Let the batter stand for 20 minutes.

3. Scoop the batter into the prepared muffin pan(s), filling each compartment about three-quarters full. (Refrigerate any remaining batter in an airtight container for up to 3 weeks.)
4. Bake for 20 to 22 minutes or until golden brown. Tops will spring back when lightly touched.

Yield: 24 muffins. Recipe easily doubles or triples. Freezes well for up to 3 months.

183 calories per muffin, 37.4 g carbohydrate, 7.1 g fiber, 4 g protein, 4.2 g fat (0.6 g saturated), 18 mg cholesterol, 235 mg sodium, 369 mg potassium, 3 mg iron, 71 mg calcium

Nutrition Notes

- *Bran Baby, Bran!* One cup of All-Bran buds with psyllium contains 39 grams of fiber whereas one cup of Bran Flakes contain just 7 grams. Natural wheat bran contains 28 grams of fiber and original All-Bran cereal contains 17.6 grams of fiber per cup. Although all are interchangeable in this recipe, go for the maximum amount of fiber for maximum health.
- *Here's the Scoop!* For even-sized muffins, use an ice cream scoop or a ⅓-cup measure, mounding the batter slightly.
- *Soy Good!* Replace ½ cup of the flour with soy flour.

Wheat Germ Bran Muffins

Wheat germ should be stored in the refrigerator to prevent it from becoming rancid.

3 tbsp tub margarine or canola oil
½ cup brown sugar, packed
¼ cup molasses
2 eggs (or 1 egg plus 2 egg whites)
1 cup skim milk

1-½ cups natural bran
¼ cup wheat germ
½ cup all-purpose flour
½ cup whole-wheat flour
1-½ tsp baking powder
½ tsp baking soda
¾ cup raisins, rinsed and drained (or chopped dates)
1 tbsp grated orange zest

1. Preheat oven to 400°F. Beat margarine with brown sugar, molasses, and eggs until well blended, about 2 or 3 minutes. Add milk and bran; blend well. Add wheat germ, flours, baking powder, and soda. Mix just until smooth. Stir in raisins and orange zest. Spoon the batter into paper-lined muffin cups, filling them about three-quarters full. Bake at 400°F for 20 to 25 minutes, until golden brown.

Yield: 12 muffins. These freeze well.

197 calories per muffin, 4.6 g fat (1 g saturated), 36 mg cholesterol, 5 g protein, 38 g carbohydrate, 223 mg sodium, 407 mg potassium, 3 mg iron, 4 g fiber, 101 mg calcium.

Variation

- **Bran and Prune Muffins:** Follow recipe for Wheat Germ Bran Muffins (page 58), but substitute 1 cup of cut-up pitted prunes for raisins. (Dip your scissors in flour first to cut prunes.)

■ SMOOTHIES

If you prefer to drink your fruit, choose a smoothie over juice—it'll provide more fiber and fewer calories. Add a tablespoon or two of ground flaxseed or wheat germ to your smoothies for additional fiber.

Chunky Monkey

Packed with potassium and fiber, plus 232 mg of calcium, what a yummy breakfast or snack!

> ¾ cup skim milk
> ½ of a frozen banana
> 1 tsp cocoa
> 2–3 ice cubes
> Sugar or sweetener to taste (2 tsp sugar or equivalent in artificial sweetener)

1.   In a blender or processor, blend the first 4 ingredients together until smooth. Add sweetener to taste.

Yield: Makes 1 serving.

155 calories per serving (with sugar), 0.9 g fat (0.5 g saturated), 3 mg cholesterol, 7 g protein, 32 g carbohydrate, 96 mg sodium, 566 mg potassium, <1 mg iron, 2 g fiber, 232 mg calcium

Fruit Smoothies

Lush slush!

> ½ cup skim milk or yogurt
> ½ cup sliced fruit (e.g., strawberries, peaches)
> ¼ tsp vanilla extract
> 2–3 ice cubes
> Sugar or sweetener to taste (1–2 tsp sugar or equivalent in artificial sweetener)

1. In a blender or processor, blend the first 4 ingredients together until smooth. Add sweetener to taste.

Yield: Makes about 1 cup.

87 calories per serving (with sugar), 0.5 g fat (0.2 g saturated), 2 mg cholesterol, 5 g protein, 16 g carbohydrate, 64 mg sodium, 343 mg potassium, trace iron, 2 g fiber, 163 mg calcium. With artificial sweetener, one serving has 74 calories and 13 g carbohydrate.

Variations

- **Banana Smoothie:** Combine ½ banana, ½ cup skim milk, ½ tsp vanilla, and 1 tsp sugar. Blend until smooth. Makes 1 serving containing about 100 calories.
- **Banana Yogurt Smoothie:** Combine 1 ripe banana, ¾ cup nonfat yogurt or buttermilk, ⅓ cup skim milk, 1 tsp honey (to taste), and 3 or 4 ice cubes. Blend until smooth. For a thicker smoothie, use a frozen banana and omit ice. Makes 2 servings.
- **Banana Strawberry Smoothie:** Combine 1 ripe banana, ½ cup sliced strawberries, ¾ cup orange or pineapple juice (or skim milk), 1 to 2 tsp honey, and 3 or 4 ice cubes. Blend until smooth. Omit ice cubes if using frozen banana or strawberries. Makes 2 servings.
- **Cantaloupe with a Banana Smoothie:** Combine the flesh of a cantaloupe, 1 banana, and 3 or 4 ice cubes. Blend until smooth. Makes 2 servings. Full of fiber and vitamins!

Mango Berry Smoothie

Dairy-free and flavorful: go man-go! If you keep frozen fruit in the freezer, you can make this 3-ingredient smoothie in a matter of seconds.

> 1 cup chopped frozen mango (or 1 mango, peeled, pitted, and cut in 1-inch chunks)
> 1 cup mixed frozen berries (try blueberries, strawberries, and/or blackberries)
> 1 cup mango, cranberry, or apple juice

1. Combine all the ingredients in a blender or food processor; blend or process until thick and creamy. If too thick, thin with a little juice or water.
2. Serve immediately or cover and refrigerate for a day or two. If you do make this ahead, shake it well before serving.

Yield: 3 servings of approximately 1 cup each.

127 calories per serving, 31.1 g carbohydrate, 3.2 g fiber, 1 g protein, 0.2 g fat (0 g saturated), 0 mg cholesterol, 25 mg sodium, 108 mg potassium, 1 mg iron, 30 mg calcium

Variations

- Instead of mango, you can substitute 1 frozen banana. I always have frozen ripe bananas on hand, so when mangoes are out of season and expensive, bananas are an economical alternative.
- Instead of berries, substitute peeled peaches, nectarines, kiwi, pineapple, or papaya, cut in chunks.
- Try pineapple, orange, pomegranate, cranberry, or guava juice as the liquid.
- Soymilk is excellent in smoothies. Just add a drizzle of honey to round out the flavor.
- *Protein Power:* To boost the protein, add 1 to 2 tbsp of whey protein powder.

■ FRUIT DISHES

Crisps and cobblers aren't just for dessert! High in fiber, they pack plenty of nutrients. Top with yogurt and serve warm on cold winter mornings.

Fabulous Fruit Crisp

This delectable dairy-free dish is very versatile. It can be baked in the oven or in the microwave, and it can be made sugar-free or nut-free without compromising its fabulous flavor. That's my kind of recipe! I keep several bags of frozen berries in my freezer so I can always prepare this dessert in minutes … and it disappears just as quickly.

Filling:
7 to 8 cups frozen mixed berries (try blueberries, strawberries, raspberries, and/or blackberries)
⅓ cup whole-wheat flour
¼ cup granulated sugar or granular Splenda
1 tsp ground cinnamon

Topping:
1 cup rolled oats (preferably large flake)
⅓ cup lightly packed brown sugar or granular Splenda
¼ cup whole-wheat flour
¼ cup sliced almonds or filberts (optional)
¼ cup canola oil or melted soft tub margarine
1 tsp ground cinnamon

1. Preheat the oven to 375°F. Combine the ingredients for the filling in a large bowl and mix well. (The berries can be added while still frozen.) Pour into a sprayed 10-inch ceramic quiche dish or 7- by 11-inch glass baking dish, and spread evenly.

63

2.   Using the same large bowl (no washing required), combine the ingredients for the topping and mix until crumbly. Sprinkle the topping over the filling in the baking dish.

3.   Bake for 40 to 45 minutes or until the topping is golden brown. To test for doneness, insert a knife into the center of the crisp. It should be hot to the touch when you remove it. Serve warm or cold.

Yield: 10 servings. Leftovers (if any) will keep for up to 3 or 4 days in the refrigerator; reheats well. Freezes well for up to 4 months.

194 calories per serving, 32.1 g carbohydrate, 4.8 g fiber, 3 g protein, 6.4 g fat (0.4 g saturated), 0 mg cholesterol, 2 mg sodium, 47 mg potassium, 2 mg iron, 32 mg calcium. If you use Splenda instead of sugar, one serving contains 162 calories and 23.8 g carbohydrate.

Variation

- **Any Kinda Crisp:** Use a total of 7 to 8 cups fruit (sliced apples, pears, peaches, plums, nectarines, strawberries, and/or rhubarb), or combine 4 cups frozen mixed berries with 3 cups frozen cubed mango. Your choice!

Chef's Secrets

- *Microwave Magic:* Place a large sheet of parchment paper under the quiche dish to catch any spills while it's baking. Microwave, uncovered, on high for 12 to 14 minutes or until the filling is bubbly and the topping is golden.
- *Double Up!* Double the recipe, using a 9- by 13-inch glass baking dish that has been sprayed with cooking spray. Bake the assembled crisp in a 375°F oven for 45 to 55 minutes. Great for a crowd.
- *Frozen Assets:* Make up batches of the topping and store it in re-sealable plastic bags in the freezer. There's no need to thaw it before using—it's ready when you are.

Jumbleberry Crisp

My cousin Nancy Gordon of Toronto gave me the idea for this fast and fabulous crisp based on her yummy Bumbleberry Pie. I combined various berries, eliminated the crust, and this delectable dish is the result. If you're missing one kind of berry, just use more of another. If using frozen berries, don't bother defrosting them. If you don't have apples, add extra berries!

Filling:
1-½ cups strawberries, hulled and sliced
2 cups blueberries
1-½ cups cranberries and/or raspberries
2 large apples, peeled, cored and sliced
⅓ cup whole-wheat flour
⅓ cup sugar (white or brown)
1 tsp cinnamon

Topping:
⅓ cup brown sugar, packed
½ cup whole-wheat flour
¾ cup quick-cooking oats
1 tsp cinnamon
¼ cup canola oil

1. Combine filling ingredients; mix well. Spray a 10-inch glass pie plate or ceramic quiche dish lightly with nonstick spray. Spread filling ingredients evenly in dish.
2. Combine topping ingredients (can be done quickly in the processor). Carefully spread topping over filling and press down slightly. Either bake at 375°F for 35 to 45 minutes until golden, or microwave uncovered on HIGH for 12 to 14 minutes, turning dish at half time. Serve hot or at room temperature. Delicious topped with a small scoop of low-fat frozen yogurt!

Yield: 10 servings. Freezes well.

202 calories per serving, 6.3 g fat (0.5 g saturated), 0 mg cholesterol, 3 g protein, 36 g carbohydrate, 6 mg sodium, 186 mg potassium, 1 mg iron, 4 g fiber, 25 mg calcium

Chef's Secrets

- Topping can be prepared ahead and frozen. No need to thaw before using!
- Prepare crisp as directed, but use 6 to 7 cups of assorted frozen berries and omit apples. Assemble in an aluminum pie plate, wrap well, and freeze it unbaked. When you need a quick dessert, unwrap the frozen crisp and bake it without defrosting at 375°F about 45 minutes.
- If you are making this dish in the microwave, place a large microsafe plate or a sheet of waxed paper under the cooking dish to catch any spills!
- *Skinny Version:* Reduce oil to 2 tbsp and add 2 tbsp water or apple juice to the topping mixture. One serving will contain 178 calories and 3.6 g fat (0.3 g saturated).
- *Skinniest Version:* Substitute 3 tbsp "lite" margarine instead of ¼ cup of oil in the topping mixture. One serving will contain 168 calories and 2.6 g fat (0.4 g saturated).
- *Fruit Crisp:* Substitute 6 to 7 cups of assorted sliced fresh (or frozen) fruits and/or berries (peaches, pears, nectarines, blackberries, etc.).

Madeleine's Fruit Clafouti

My lighter version of her French pudding-like dish made with peaches, plums, pears, or berries.

3 cups fresh fruit of your choice (e.g., peaches)
2 tbsp plus ¼ cup sugar
1 cup skim milk
1 cup nonfat yogurt
2 eggs plus 2 egg whites (or 3 eggs)
½ cup flour
⅛ tsp salt
1 tsp vanilla

1. Preheat oven to 375°F. Spray a 2-quart baking dish with nonstick spray. Arrange sliced, peeled fruit in dish; sprinkle with 2 tbsp sugar. Combine remaining ingredients in processor. Process for 45 seconds, until smooth. Pour batter over fruit and bake for 45 to 50 minutes, until browned.

Yield: 8 servings. Delicious served warm or at room temperature.

145 calories per serving, 1.6 g fat (0.5 g saturated), 54 mg cholesterol, 7 g protein, 27 g carbohydrate, 118 mg sodium, 292 mg potassium, <1 mg iron, 2 g fiber, 110 mg calcium

Chef's Secret
- Use whole-wheat pastry flour to boost the fiber content.

Peachy Crumb Crisp

Filling:
6 cups peeled, sliced peaches (or a combination of peaches, nectarines, and plums)
1 tbsp lemon juice
¼ cup brown sugar, packed
¼ cup whole-wheat flour
1 tsp cinnamon

Topping:
¼ cup brown sugar, packed
½ cup whole-wheat flour
¾ cup quick-cooking oats
1 tsp cinnamon
2 tbsp tub margarine or canola oil
2 tbsp orange juice

1. Combine filling ingredients and place in a sprayed 10-inch ceramic quiche dish. Combine topping ingredients and mix until crumbly. Sprinkle over fruit. Bake at 400°F for 45 minutes. If necessary, cover loosely with foil to prevent overbrowning.

Yield: 10 servings. Freezes well.

162 calories per serving, 2.9 g fat (0.5 g saturated), 0 mg cholesterol, 3 g protein, 33 g carbohydrate, 24 mg sodium, 308 mg potassium, 1 mg iron, 4 g fiber, 27 mg calcium

Variations

- **Blueberry Peach Crisp:** Use 4 cups sliced peaches and 2 cups blueberries in the filling. Add 1 tsp grated orange zest.
- **Blueberry Nectarine Crisp:** Use 4 cups sliced nectarines and 2 cups blueberries in the filling.
- **Apple Crisp:** Instead of peaches, use 6 cups sliced apples. Add ½ tsp nutmeg.
- **Strawberry Rhubarb Crisp:** Instead of peaches, use 2 cups sliced strawberries and 4 cups fresh or frozen (thawed) rhubarb, cut in ½-inch pieces. Increase sugar in filling to ⅔ cup. Add 1 tsp grated orange zest.

CHAPTER FIVE

LUNCH

WHAT'S INSIDE

■ SOUPS

Bean and vegetable soups are loaded with fiber. They withstand the freezer well, so you can make a big batch, freeze in containers, and bring to work for quick and healthy lunches.

Autumn Vegetable Soup

This scrumptious low-cal, low-carb autumn soup is wonderful any time of year. The recipe comes from Valerie Kanter of Chicago, editor of the Kosher cookbook *Crowning Elegance*. Her family loves it, especially her children, who devour two or three bowlfuls at one sitting. Valerie often serves it from her slow cooker for the Sabbath lunch. It's a winner!

2 tbsp olive oil
1 large onion, chopped
2 to 3 stalks celery, chopped
6 medium carrots (1 lb/500 g), peeled and chopped
3 medium sweet potatoes, peeled and cut in chunks
1 medium butternut or acorn squash, peeled and cut in chunks (about 5 cups)
1 cup sliced mushrooms
2 medium zucchini, cut in chunks
10 cups water
4 to 6 bay leaves
1 tbsp salt (or to taste)
½ tsp freshly ground black pepper
2 tbsp finely chopped fresh dillweed
2 tbsp finely chopped fresh parsley
1 clove garlic (about 1 tsp minced)

1. Heat the oil in a large soup pot on medium heat. Sauté the onion, celery, and carrots for 5 minutes or until the vegetables are tender, stirring occasionally. Add the sweet potatoes, squash, mushrooms, and zucchini; mix well.

2. Add the water, bay leaves, salt, and pepper, and bring to a boil. Reduce heat to low and simmer, partially covered, for 2 hours, stirring occasionally. If the soup becomes too thick, add a little more water. Remove the bay leaves and discard.

3. Using a potato masher, coarsely mash the vegetables while still in the pot, leaving the soup somewhat chunky. Stir in the dillweed, parsley, and garlic. Serve hot.

Yield: 8 to 10 servings (about 15 cups). Keeps for up to 3 to 4 days in the refrigerator; reheats well.

78 calories per cup, 15.1 g carbohydrate, 3.8 g fiber, 1 g protein, 2.0 g fat (0.3 saturated), 0 mg cholesterol, 548 mg sodium, 443 mg potassium, 1 mg iron, 46 mg calcium

Chef's Secrets

- *Short Cuts:* To make it easier to cut a squash, slash the tough outer skin in several places with a sharp knife. Microwave, uncovered, on high for 4 to 5 minutes. Cool for 5 minutes, then cut in half or in large pieces. Remove the seeds and stringy fibers—an ice-cream scoop works perfectly.
- *Love Me Tender!* Summer squash varieties include zucchini, crookneck, and patty-pan squash—all have thin, edible skins and soft seeds. Summer squash cooks quickly because of the high water content.
- *Bay Watch!* Always remove and discard bay leaves after cooking. A bay leaf won't rehydrate even after boiling, so if left in the soup, someone could choke on it. Count how many you put in and how many you take out. Or, better yet, tie them up in a square of cheesecloth for easy removal after cooking.

Bean, Barley and Sweet Potato Soup

1 cup dried white beans (navy or pea)
3 cups cold water
2 tsp canola or olive oil
2 large onions, peeled and chopped
4 stalks celery, trimmed and chopped
2 zucchini, chopped (optional)
1 red pepper, chopped (optional)
8 cups chicken broth or hot water
4 carrots, sliced
1 sweet potato, peeled and chopped
½ cup pearl barley, rinsed and drained
½ tsp pepper
1 tsp dried basil
Salt, to taste

1. Soak beans in water overnight. Drain and rinse well. Discard soaking water. Heat oil on medium heat in a large heavy-bottomed soup pot. Sauté onions and celery for 5 minutes, until golden. Add zucchini and red pepper and cook 5 minutes longer. Add a little water if needed to prevent burning. Add remaining ingredients except salt. Bring to a boil. Reduce heat, cover partially and simmer for 2 hours, stirring occasionally. If soup is too thick, add a little water. Add salt; season to taste.

Yield: 10 to 12 servings.

173 calories per serving, 1.3 g fat (0.2 g saturated), 0 mg cholesterol, 12 g protein, 29 g carbohydrate, 175 mg sodium, 498 mg potassium, 4 mg iron, 7 g fiber, 90 mg calcium

Black Bean Soup

Excellent, easy, and full of fiber! Impress your guests with its wonderful South American flavor.

2 cups dried black beans, rinsed and drained
6 cups cold water (for soaking the beans)
2 onions, coarsely chopped
4 cloves garlic, minced
4 stalks celery, coarsely chopped
1 tbsp olive oil
4 large carrots, coarsely chopped
1 tsp dried basil
½ tsp dried red pepper flakes
1 tsp cumin (to taste)
8 cups chicken or vegetable broth (about)
Salt and pepper, to taste

1. Soak beans overnight in cold water. Drain and rinse well. Discard soaking water.
2. Prepare vegetables. (This can be done in the processor.) Heat oil in a large soup pot. Add onions, garlic and celery. Sauté for 5 or 6 minutes on medium heat, until golden. If necessary, add a little water or broth to prevent sticking.
3. Add drained beans, carrots, seasonings and broth. Do not add salt and pepper until beans are cooked. Cover partially and simmer until beans are tender, about 2 hours, stirring occasionally. Purée part or all of the soup, if desired. If too thick, thin with water or broth. Add salt and pepper to taste.

Yield: 10 servings.

188 calories per serving, 2.1 g fat (0.3 g saturated), 0 mg cholesterol, 14 g protein, 29 g carbohydrate, 171 mg sodium, 495 mg potassium, 4 mg iron, 10 g fiber, 69 mg calcium

Chef's Secrets

- Soak and drain beans as directed in Step 1. Place soaked beans in a storage container and pop them in the freezer for up to 2 months. When you want to make soup, just add the frozen beans to the pot. No need to defrost them first. (You can use this trick with any kind of beans!) P.S. Don't add salt to your soup until navy or kidney beans are almost done. Otherwise, they'll never get soft! However, if using lima beans, you can add salt at the beginning of cooking without any problem.
- If you have time, presoak a batch of black beans, then cook them for 1-½ to 2 hours, until tender. Drain, cool, and freeze. When you want soup, add 3 to 4 cups of frozen cooked beans to the soup pot without thawing. Your soup will be ready in just half an hour!
- If you're really in a rush, substitute two 14 oz (398 ml) cans of black beans, drained and rinsed, instead of soaking dried beans overnight. Cooking time with canned beans is also half an hour.
- Are you afraid to eat beans because you're worried about possible embarrassing moments? If you presoak beans, then discard the soaking water, you'll also eliminate the problem of gas! As an extra precaution, rinse the beans again thoroughly after presoaking them.
- *Serving Tip:* For an elegant touch, garnish each serving with a swirl of nonfat yogurt. If necessary, thin yogurt with a little milk. Use a plastic squeeze bottle to squeeze a design with the yogurt. Top with a spoonful of bottled or homemade salsa.

Broccoli and Red Pepper Soup

Broccoli rocks in this stalk-filled soup! This low-cal, low-carb soup is a light "weigh" to start a meal and curb your appetite.

1 tbsp olive oil
1 medium onion, chopped
1 red pepper, seeded and chopped
2 cloves garlic (about 2 tsp minced)

2 carrots, coarsely chopped (or 12 baby carrots)

1 bunch broccoli, trimmed and coarsely chopped (about 4 cups)

6 cups vegetable broth

1 to 2 tsp salt (or to taste)

½ tsp freshly ground black pepper

1 tsp dried basil or 1 tbsp chopped fresh basil

3 tbsp chopped fresh dillweed

Light sour cream, nonfat yogurt, or skim milk (optional)

1. Heat the oil in a large saucepan on medium heat. Add the onion, red pepper, and garlic, and sauté for 3 to 4 minutes or until the vegetables are tender. Stir in the carrots and broccoli and mix well.

2. Add the broth, salt, pepper, basil, and dillweed, and bring to a boil. Reduce heat and simmer, partially covered, for 20 minutes or until the broccoli is tender. Remove from heat and cool slightly.

3. Using an immersion blender, purée the soup while still in the pot, or purée in batches in a blender or food processor. Adjust the seasonings to taste and serve with a dollop of sour cream, yogurt, or a little milk, if desired.

Yield: 4 to 6 servings (about 8 cups). Keeps 3 to 4 days in the refrigerator; reheats well. Freezes well for up to 4 months.

84 calories per cup, 13.7 g carbohydrate, 3.7 g fiber, 3 g protein, 2.4 g fat (0.3 g saturated), 0 mg cholesterol, 527 mg sodium, 354 mg potassium, 1 mg iron, 67 mg calcium

Nutrition Notes

- This scrumptious soup is high in fiber, potassium, beta carotene, and vitamins A and C.
- Frozen broccoli, which is mostly florets, may actually contain more beta carotene than fresh broccoli. Add fresh or frozen broccoli florets to this nutritious soup. The stems from fresh broccoli can be grated and used instead of cabbage when making stir-fries or coleslaw.

Easy Corn Chowder

In the summertime, make this chunky soup with fresh corn and in the winter, use frozen. Corn and broccoli are excellent sources of lutein, which helps keep your eyes healthy … so, the "eyes" have it!

1 tbsp extra virgin olive oil
2 medium onions, chopped
2 stalks celery, chopped
1 red pepper, seeded and chopped
4 cups fresh (about 6 ears) or frozen corn kernels
1 medium potato, peeled (about 1 cup chopped)
2 cups broccoli florets
3 cups vegetable broth
1 tsp salt
½ tsp freshly ground black pepper
½ tsp dried thyme
1 tsp dried basil or 2 tbsp chopped fresh basil
1 cup skim milk or soymilk

1. Heat the oil in a large saucepan on medium heat. Add the onions, celery, and red pepper, and sauté for 5 minutes or until the vegetables are tender. Add the corn and potato and cook 4 to 5 minutes longer, stirring often.
2. Add the broccoli, broth, salt, pepper, and thyme (if using dried basil, add it now), and bring to a boil. Reduce heat to low, cover, and simmer for 10 to 12 minutes or until the potatoes are tender. Remove from heat and cool slightly. If using fresh basil, add it now.
3. Using an immersion blender, partially purée the soup while still in the pot (or purée half the vegetables with a little of the cooking liquid in a food processor or blender and then return the purée to the pot). Add the milk and reheat gently on low heat. Don't bring to a boil or the soup may curdle.

Yield: 5 to 6 servings (about 7 cups). Keeps for up to 3 to 4 days in the refrigerator; reheats well. Freezes well for up to 3 months. If soup is too thick, add a little milk or soymilk.

112 calories per cup, 22.5 g carbohydrate, 3.5 g fiber, 4 g protein, 2.1 g fat (0.3 g saturated), 0 mg cholesterol, 339 mg sodium, 327 mg potassium, 1 mg iron, 49 mg calcium

Chef's Secrets
- *Ears to You!* If using fresh corn, remove the husks and silk. (A damp paper towel removes the silk quickly.) Cut the ears in half crosswise with a sharp knife, then stand each piece on its cut end and slice downward several times to cut off all the kernels. One ear yields about ¾ cup corn kernels.
- *Green Cuisine!* Instead of broccoli, add 2 cups frozen green peas. Instead of onions, substitute 2 leeks, using the white and light green parts.

Luscious Lentil Soup

Easy and healthy! Although it takes about the same amount of time to microwave this soup as to cook it on top of the stove, it never sticks to the bottom of the pot when you microwave it. Your food processor will chop the vegetables 1-2-3.

1 large onion, chopped
4 cloves garlic, minced
1 tbsp olive or canola oil
1 cup brown or red lentils, rinsed and drained
1 stalk celery, chopped
28 oz (796 ml) can tomatoes (or 5 to 6 fresh ripe tomatoes, chopped)
5 cups water (approximately)
1 bay leaf
1-½ tsp salt (to taste)
½ tsp pepper
1 tsp dried basil or dill (or 1 tbsp fresh)
Juice of half a lemon (1–½ tbsp)
¼ cup parsley, minced

1.   *Microwave Method:* In a 3-quart microsafe pot, combine onion, garlic, and oil. Microwave uncovered on HIGH for 4 minutes. Add remaining ingredients except lemon juice and parsley; mix well. Microwave covered on HIGH for 1 hour, until lentils are tender. Stir once or twice during cooking. If boiling too much, reduce power to MEDIUM (50%). If too thick, add some boiling water. Add lemon juice. Adjust seasonings to taste. Let stand at least 10 minutes to allow flavors to blend. Discard bay leaf. Garnish with parsley.

2.   *Conventional Method:* Heat oil in a large soup pot. Add onions; sauté on medium heat until golden, about 4 or 5 minutes. Add garlic and sauté 2 or 3 minutes longer. Add 2 or 3 tablespoons of water if vegetables begin to stick. Add remaining ingredients except lemon juice and parsley. Bring to a boil, reduce heat and simmer 1 hour, until lentils are tender, stirring occasionally. Thin with a little hot water if too thick. Add lemon juice. Adjust seasonings to taste. Discard bay leaf. Garnish with parsley.

Yield: 8 to 10 servings. Tastes even better the next day!

120 calories per serving, 2.1 g fat (0.3 g saturated), 0 mg cholesterol, 7 g protein, 20 g carbohydrate, 603 mg sodium, 533 mg potassium, 3 mg iron, 7 g fiber, 63 mg calcium

Variations

- For more fiber, add 2 or 3 carrots, coarsely chopped, to the sautéed onions. Proceed as directed. Add 1 cup of cooked pasta or rice to the cooked soup, or sprinkle with a little grated Parmesan cheese. For a Middle Eastern flavor, substitute coriander (cilantro) for basil or dill.
- **Lentil, Vegetable and Barley Soup:** Prepare Luscious Lentil Soup as directed above, but add 3 potatoes, 3 carrots, and 1 zucchini, coarsely chopped, to the sautéed vegetables. Also add ⅓ cup barley, which has been rinsed and drained. Then continue as directed. If cooked soup is too thick, add a little water or vegetable stock.

Mighty Minestrone

This quick and easy fiber-filled soup comes from my cousin Elsie Gorewich. It was a favorite of her late daughter Nancy, who included the recipe in her cookbook *Souperb!* Every year Nancy compiled a small cookbook that she sent to family and friends. I'm so glad I have my own copy, which is part of my treasured cookbook collection.

2 tbsp olive oil
2 to 3 cloves garlic (about 2 to 3 tsp minced)
2 stalks celery, chopped
2 medium carrots, chopped
1 medium onion, chopped
1 can (28 oz/796 ml) whole tomatoes, undrained
1 can (19 oz/540 ml) red kidney beans, drained and rinsed
3 medium zucchini, chopped
2 cups vegetable or chicken broth
1 tsp dried oregano
Salt and freshly ground black pepper
Pinch of sugar (optional)
Chopped fresh basil, for garnish

1. Heat the oil in a large soup pot on medium heat. Add the garlic, celery, carrots, and onion; sauté until tender, about 5 minutes. Add the tomatoes, kidney beans, zucchini, broth, and oregano; bring to a boil. Reduce heat and simmer, partially covered, for 25 to 30 minutes. Stir occasionally. If the soup becomes too thick, thin with a little broth or water.
2. Season with salt and pepper. If necessary, add a pinch of sugar. (Some brands of canned tomatoes are more acidic than others; a small amount of sugar will counter than acidity.) Garnish with fresh basil and serve.

Yield: 6 to 8 servings (about 10 cups). Keeps 3 to 4 days in the refrigerator; reheats well. Freezes well for up to 4 months.

117 calories per cup, 19.2 g carbohydrate, 5.7 g fiber, 4 g protein, 3.2 g fat (0.4 g saturated), 0 mg cholesterol, 481 mg sodium, 500 mg potassium, 2 mg iron, 66 mg calcium

Variations

- Instead of zucchini, substitute green or yellow beans, trimmed and cut in 1-inch pieces. For a calcium boost, add a sprinkling of grated Parmesan cheese or a dollop of low-fat sour cream at serving time.

Chef's Secrets

- *Machine Cuisine!* Chop the vegetables in batches in the food processor, using quick on/off pulses.
- *Microwave Magic!* Combine the oil, garlic, celery, carrots, and onion in a 3-quart microwaveable pot. Microwave, covered, on high for 5 minutes. Add the remaining ingredients and microwave, covered, on high for 20 minutes, stirring once or twice.

Quick Pea Soup

This fabulous, fiber-filled soup, which uses frozen peas, is sure to "ap-pease" your hunger. The original recipe came from Sandra Gitlin, who is a superb cook. I substituted spinach for iceberg lettuce, added garlic and fresh basil, and reduced the cooking time from 1-½ hours to just 30 minutes to retain more nutrients.

4 tsp olive oil
1 large onion, sliced
4 cups lightly packed baby spinach leaves
2 medium carrots, cut in chunks
1 medium potato, peeled and cut in chunks
1 pkg (2 lb/1 kg) frozen green sweet peas or baby peas (no need to defrost)
8 cups vegetable broth

3 to 4 cloves garlic (about 1 tbsp minced)

2 tsp curry powder or 1 tsp ground cumin

1 tsp salt (or to taste)

½ tsp freshly ground black pepper

3 to 4 tbsp minced fresh basil

1. Heat the oil in a large soup pot on medium heat. Add the onion and sauté for about 5 to 7 minutes or until golden.

2. Add the remaining ingredients, except the basil, to the soup pot and bring to a boil. Reduce heat to low and simmer, partially covered, for 30 minutes or until the vegetables are tender. Remove from heat and cool slightly.

3. Using an immersion blender, purée the soup while still in the pot, or purée in batches in a blender or food processor. Stir in the basil and adjust the seasonings to taste.

Yield: 6 to 8 servings (about 11 cup). Keeps 3 to 4 days in the refrigerator; reheats well. Freezes well for up to 4 months.

117 calories per cup, 19.3 g carbohydrate, 6.5 g fiber, 6 g protein, 2.3 g fat (0.3 g saturated), 0 mg cholesterol, 626 mg sodium, 217 mg potassium, 2 mg iron, 53 mg calcium

Chef's Secrets

- *Frozen Assets:* Most people keep green peas in their freezer. Frozen peas have additional benefits besides acting as an ice pack. One-half cup of frozen peas contains 62 calories, 11.4 g carbohydrate, 4.4 g fiber, and 4 grams of protein, plus they're virtually fat-free.

- *Sodi-Yum!* If you are concerned about sodium, use a salt-free vegetable broth.

- *Dairy Delicious!* For a calcium boost, add a swirl of yogurt or a dollop of low-fat sour cream at serving time.

Red Lentil, Zucchini and Couscous Soup

1 large onion, chopped
1 stalk celery, chopped
2 tsp olive oil
3–4 carrots, grated
2 medium zucchini, grated
1 cup red lentils, picked over, rinsed and drained
6 cups water or vegetable broth (about)
2 tsp salt (or to taste)
½ tsp pepper
½ tsp dried basil
⅓ cup couscous

1. Onions and celery can be chopped in the processor, using quick on/off turns. Heat oil in a 5-quart soup pot. Add onions and celery. Sauté on medium-high heat for 5 to 7 minutes, or until golden. If vegetables begin to stick, add a tablespoon or two of water.
2. Meanwhile, grate carrots and zucchini. Add all ingredients except couscous to pot. Bring to a boil. Reduce heat and simmer partially covered for 45 minutes, stirring occasionally. Add couscous and simmer 10 minutes longer. If soup is too thick, thin with a little water. Adjust seasonings to taste.

Yield: 8 servings.

134 calories per serving, 1.5 g fat (0.2 g saturated), 0 mg cholesterol, 8 g protein, 24 g carbohydrate, 612 mg sodium, 430 mg potassium, 3 mg iron, 8 g fiber, 39 mg calcium

■ SALADS AND DRESSINGS

Though lettuce salads contain little fiber, there are plenty of vegetable and grain salads that really pack it in. Many of them make excellent to-go lunches.

Apricot Hoisin Spinach Salad

Apricot Hoisin Marinade, an Asian delight, is reinvented as a salad dressing with the addition of orange juice and oil, then is served over a fiber-packed combination of almonds, apricots, snow peas, and spinach or mixed greens. You can transform this marvelous Asian salad into a main dish by simply adding a scoop of chicken, tuna, or salmon salad.

Dressing:
½ cup Apricot Hoisin Marinade (page 279)
¼ cup orange juice (preferably fresh)
1 tsp canola oil

Salad:
1 bag (10 oz/300 g) baby spinach leaves or mixed salad greens
1 red pepper, seeded and cut into strips
½ red onion, thinly sliced
½ cup grated carrots
2 cups snow peas, trimmed
1 cup sliced dried apricots
½ cup toasted sliced almonds or sesame seeds, for garnish

1. In a small bowl, whisk together ingredients for the dressing and blend well. Set aside.
2. In a large bowl, combine the spinach, red pepper, onion, carrots, snow peas, and apricots. (If desired, the vegetables and dressing can be prepared in advance up to this point and refrigerated separately for several hours.)
3. At serving time, combine the salad ingredients with the dressing and toss gently to mix. Top with almonds and serve immediately.

Yield: 6 servings. Dressing keeps for up to a week in the refrigerator.

180 calories per serving, 31.2 g carbohydrate, 6.3 g fiber, 5 g protein, 5.8 g fat (0.5 g saturated), 0 mg cholesterol, 242 mg sodium, 477 mg potassium, 3 mg iron, 86 mg calcium

Variation

- **Apricot Hoisin Chicken and Spinach Salad:** Marinate 4 to 6 boneless, skinless chicken breasts in ½ to ¾ cup Apricot Hoisin Marinade for 30 minutes; grill for 5 to 6 minutes per side. When cool, slice chicken thinly and arrange attractively on top of salad. So chic!

Balsamic Vinaigrette

This simple, versatile dressing is scrumptious on salads or can be used to marinate chicken, fish, or roasted vegetables. When you make your own salad dressings, you can control the sodium content and choose healthier fats such as extra virgin olive oil. You won't regret making this vinaigrette.

1 clove garlic (about 1 tsp minced)
¼ cup balsamic vinegar
½ cup extra virgin olive oil
2 tsp maple syrup or honey
¼ tsp salt
Freshly ground black pepper
¼ tsp each dried basil and thyme

1. Combine all the ingredients in a jar, cover tightly, and shake well. Store in the refrigerator until ready to use. Shake well before using.

Yield: About ¾ cup. Keeps for up to 2 to 3 months in the refrigerator.

86 calories per tbsp, 1.5 g carbohydrate, 0 g fiber, 0 g protein, 8.8 g fat (1.2 g saturated), 0 mg cholesterol, 47 mg sodium, 8 mg potassium, 0 mg iron, 3 mg calcium

Best Green Bean Salad

This outstanding salad is served in many popular Greek restaurants. It's become my favorite way to eat green beans because it's absolutely delicious! This recipe also works well with yellow wax beans.

1 lb (500 g) green beans
8 cups water
Salt
½ red pepper, chopped
2 green onions, chopped
¼ cup minced fresh dillweed
2 tbsp lemon juice (preferably fresh)
2 tbsp extra virgin olive oil
Coarse salt and freshly ground black pepper

1. Snap off both ends from each green bean; rinse well. Meanwhile, bring the water, sprinkled with salt, to a boil in a large pot. Add the beans and cook, uncovered, for 3 to 4 minutes or just until tender-crisp and bright green. Drain immediately. Rinse the beans under cold water to stop the cooking process. Drain well and set aside to cool completely.
2. Combine the cooled green beans with the red pepper, green onions, and dillweed in a large bowl, cover, and refrigerate until serving time.
3. When ready to serve, add the lemon juice and olive oil to the green beans. Season with salt and pepper to taste and toss to combine. Serve immediately.

Yield: 4 to 6 servings. Leftovers keep for up to 1 to 2 days in the refrigerator, but the color won't be as vibrant.

110 calories per serving, 10.9 g carbohydrate, 4.1 g fiber, 2 g protein, 7.4 g fat (1.1 g saturated), 0 mg cholesterol, 268 mg sodium, 228 mg potassium, 1 mg iron, 57 mg calcium

Chef's Secrets

- *Less-Than-7 Rule:* To preserve their bright color, cook green beans and other green vegetables for no more than 7 minutes. Plunging green vegetables in ice cold water immediately after cooking them stops the cooking process and preserves their color.
- *Buffet Beauty:* For a large crowd, double or triple the recipe and serve it on a large serving platter. Top with crumbled feta cheese.
- *No dillweed?* Substitute chopped fresh basil.

Carrot Almond Salad

This quick-to-make, tasty, and brightly colored salad has eye appeal—now you see it, but soon you won't!

> 1 bag (10 oz/283 g) grated carrots (about 3 cups)
> 2 green onions, thinly sliced
> ½ cup dried cranberries or raisins
> ½ cup toasted slivered almonds
> 2 tbsp extra virgin olive oil
> 2 tbsp lemon juice (preferably fresh) or vinegar
> 1 tbsp honey or granular Splenda
> 1 tsp Dijon mustard
> 2 tbsp minced fresh dillweed or parsley
> ½ tsp salt

1. In a large bowl, combine the carrots, green onions, cranberries, and almonds.
2. In a small bowl, whisk together the oil, lemon juice, honey, mustard, dillweed, and salt. Drizzle over the carrot mixture and mix well. Cover and refrigerate for up to 1 to 2 hours or overnight, before serving.

Yield: 6 servings. Recipe doubles and triples easily. Keeps for up to 2 to 3 days in the refrigerator.

*162 calories per serving, 18.7 g carbohydrate, 3.1 g fiber, 3 g protein, 9.4 g fat (1.0 g saturated), 0 mg cholesterol, 249 mg sodium, 255 mg potassium, 1 mg iron, 46 mg calcium. **Nutrition Note**—Sweet Choice! With Splenda, one serving contains 152 calories and 16.0 g carbohydrate.*

Couscous, Cranberry and Mango Salad

This colorful, low-fat salad comes together quickly—no cooking required!

1-½ cups hot vegetable or chicken broth
1 cup whole-wheat couscous
½ cup fresh parsley or ¼ cup fresh mint
2 tbsp chopped fresh basil
1 slice fresh ginger, peeled (about 1 tbsp minced)
2 cloves garlic (about 2 tsp minced)
3 green onions or ½ cup chopped red onion
1 red pepper
½ cup dried cranberries
1 large ripe mango, peeled and diced

Dressing:
2 tbsp soy sauce (low-sodium or regular)
2 tbsp rice vinegar
1 tbsp Asian (toasted) sesame oil
1 tbsp orange juice (preferably fresh)
Freshly ground black pepper

1. Combine the hot broth with couscous in a large bowl. Cover and let stand 10 minutes, until the liquid is absorbed. Fluff with a fork.
2. In a food processor fitted with the steel blade, process the parsley, basil, ginger, and garlic until minced, about 10 seconds. Add to the couscous. Cut the green onions and red pepper into chunks. Process with quick on/ off pulses, until coarsely chopped. Add to the couscous along with the dried cranberries and mango.

3. Add the soy sauce, vinegar, sesame oil, orange juice, and pepper to couscous; mix gently to combine. (If desired, this salad can be prepared a day in advance and refrigerated.) Adjust the seasonings to taste before serving.

Yield: 8 servings (about ½ cup each). Recipe doubles and triples easily. Keeps for up to 2 to 3 days in the refrigerator.

128 calories per serving, 25.8 g carbohydrate, 3.4 g fiber, 3 g protein, 2.3 g fat (0.3 g saturated), 0 mg cholesterol, 211 mg sodium, 131 mg potassium, 1 mg iron, 25 mg calcium

Variations
- Instead of mango, use 1 cup fresh pineapple or oranges, cut into bite-sized pieces. Add some diced celery, water chestnuts, and/or bamboo shoots for extra crunch. Garnish with toasted sliced almonds or chopped pistachios.

Creamy 1,000 Island Cole Slaw
This super slaw is virtually fat-free and high in fiber and potassium. Enjoy without guilt!

1 medium green cabbage (about 8 cups shredded)
6 green onions, chopped
3 stalks celery, chopped
1 green and 1 red pepper, chopped
3 carrots, grated
½ cup nonfat yogurt
½ cup nonfat or low-fat mayonnaise
½ cup ketchup or salsa
2 tbsp fresh chopped basil (or 1 tsp dried)
2 tbsp minced fresh dill
Salt and pepper, to taste

1. Prepare vegetables. (You can do this quickly in the processor.) Combine veggies in a large bowl. Add remaining ingredients; mix well. Chill to blend flavors.

Yield: 12 servings. Leftovers will keep for several days in the refrigerator.

50 calories per serving, 0.3 g fat (0 g saturated), trace cholesterol, 2 g protein, 11 g carbohydrate, 225 mg sodium, 326 mg potassium, <1 mg iron, 3 g fiber, 60 mg calcium

Variation

- *Non-Dairy Version:* Omit yogurt, mayonnaise, and ketchup. Substitute 1-½ cups bottled low-calorie 1,000 Island salad dressing. If desired, fold in 1 cup of drained pineapple tidbits.

Doug's "Flower Power" Cæsar Salad

This super salad is nutrient-packed. It's a specialty of my son Doug, the Salad King!

    3 cups broccoli florets
    3 cups cauliflower florets
    1 cup sliced red cabbage
    3 tbsp grated Parmesan cheese
    ¾ cup Lighter Cæsar Salad Dressing (page 96) or bottled low-fat Cæsar
        dressing
    ½ tsp freshly ground pepper

1. Wash vegetables well; drain thoroughly. Combine all ingredients in a glass bowl and mix well. (Optional: Steam the veggies for 3 or 4 minutes if you prefer them softer.) This salad keeps for 3 days in a glass (not metal) bowl in the refrigerator, if well-covered.

Yield: 6 servings.

68 calories per serving, 2.2 g fat (1.4 g saturated), 6 mg cholesterol, 6 g protein, 8 g carbohydrate, 401 mg sodium, 348 mg potassium, <1 mg iron, 3 g fiber, 148 mg calcium

Fattouche Salad

A fresh and lemony Middle Eastern salad. Toasted pita is added just before serving. Yummy!

2 medium pitas
1 bunch flat-leaf or curly parsley
1 head iceberg or romaine lettuce
2–3 ripe tomatoes, diced
½ of an English cucumber, diced
4 green onions (or 1 small onion, diced)

Dressing:
Juice of 1 lemon (3 tbsp)
2 tbsp fresh mint, finely chopped
3–4 tbsp olive oil (preferably extra virgin)
1 clove garlic, crushed (optional)
Salt and pepper, to taste

1. Split pitas in half and place on an ungreased baking sheet. Bake in a preheated 400°F oven until crisp, about 10 minutes. Break pitas into small pieces and set aside. Wash parsley and lettuce; dry well. Mince parsley leaves; tear lettuce in bite-sized pieces. In a large bowl, combine lettuce, parsley, tomatoes, cucumber and onions; chill. Combine dressing ingredients; set aside. Just before serving, combine all ingredients and mix well. Serve immediately.

Yield: 6 servings. Leftover salad will become soggy.

150 calories per serving, 7.7 g fat (1.1 g saturated), 0 mg cholesterol, 4 g protein, 18 g carbohydrate, 127 mg sodium, 386 mg potassium, 2 mg iron, 3 g fiber, 62 mg calcium

Greek Chickpea Salad

This tasty salad comes from Debbie Morson, of Toronto, who assisted with some of the recipe testing for this book. It's full of fiber, flavor, and phytochemicals, making it an excellent vegetarian dish.

1 can (19 oz/540 ml) chickpeas, drained and rinsed
1 red or yellow pepper, seeded and chopped
1 green pepper, seeded and chopped
1 cup chopped sweet onion (try Vidalia)
¾ of an English cucumber, unpeeled, halved, seeded, and chopped
1 medium tomato, chopped
¼ cup minced fresh basil
2 tbsp minced fresh dillweed
1 clove garlic (about 1 tsp minced)
Juice of 1 lemon (about 3 tbsp)
3 tbsp extra virgin olive oil
½ to ¾ cup pitted and halved black olives
Salt and freshly ground black pepper
½ cup crumbled light feta cheese

1. Place the drained chickpeas in a large bowl. Add the peppers, onion, cucumber, tomato, basil, dillweed, and garlic; mix well. Add the lemon juice, olive oil, olives, salt, and pepper to taste; toss gently to mix. Crumble the feta cheese over the top, cover, and chill before serving.
2. When ready to serve, adjust seasonings and drain off any excess liquid.

Yield: 8 servings. Keeps for up to 2 to 3 days in the refrigerator.

177 calories per serving, 20.2 g carbohydrate, 4.1 g fiber, 7 g protein, 8.5 g fat (2.0 g saturated), 5 mg cholesterol, 440 mg sodium, 266 mg potassium, 1 mg iron, 67 mg calcium

Indonesian Brown Rice Salad

This addictive rice salad was my favorite dish at a pot luck birthday party. Suzi Lipes generously shared this wonderful recipe with me; I reduced the fat and now share it with you. It's a winner!

1 cup brown rice
2 cups boiling water
½ cup raisins
2 cups green onions, chopped
1 cup fresh bean sprouts
1 red pepper, chopped
1 stalk celery, chopped
¼ cup toasted sesame seeds
¼ cup toasted pecans, chopped (optional)

Salad Dressing:
⅓ cup fresh orange juice
3–4 tbsp canola or olive oil
1 tbsp Oriental sesame oil
¼ cup tamari or low-sodium soy sauce
2 tbsp sherry
2 cloves garlic, finely minced (about 1 tsp)
½-inch slice ginger, finely minced
Freshly ground pepper, to taste

1. Combine rice and boiling water in a saucepan. Cover, bring to a boil, and simmer for 30 minutes. Remove from heat and let cool. Meanwhile, prepare remaining ingredients. Salad dressing can be prepared in the processor. In a large bowl, combine all ingredients except sesame seeds and pecans. Mix well. Cover and refrigerate for several hours or overnight to blend flavors. At serving time, add sesame seeds and pecans.

Yield: 8 servings as a side dish, or 10 to 12 servings as part of a buffet.

232 calories per serving, 9.7 g fat (1.1 g saturated), 0 mg cholesterol, 5 g protein, 33 g carbohydrate, 542 mg sodium, 302 mg potassium, 2 mg iron, 4 g fiber, 46 mg calcium

Israeli Salad

I love to cook, but don't always have the patience to chop vegetables into the small cubes that make this salad so delicious. Bring a small taste of Israel to your table! This is a favorite at a buffet. Recipe can be halved, if desired.

> 1 head of romaine or iceberg lettuce
> 4 green onions
> 1 medium onion
> 2 green peppers
> 1 red pepper
> 1 English cucumber, peeled
> 8 firm, ripe tomatoes (preferably Israeli)
> 4 tbsp olive oil (preferably extra virgin)
> 4 tbsp fresh lemon juice
> 1 tsp salt (or to taste)
> Freshly ground pepper, optional

1. Wash and dry vegetables well. Dice them neatly into ½-inch pieces and combine in a large bowl. Sprinkle with olive oil and lemon juice. Add seasonings; mix again. Adjust seasonings to taste.

Yield: 8 servings. Salad tastes best eaten the same day it is made, but leftovers will keep for a day in the refrigerator. Drain off excess liquid in the bottom of the bowl before serving.

127 calories per serving, 7.7 g fat (1.1 g saturated), 0 mg cholesterol, 3 g protein, 14 g carbohydrate, 600 mg sodium, 637 mg potassium, 2 mg iron, 4 g fiber, 45 mg calcium

Variation

- **Mediterranean Vegetable Salad:** Add ½ cup sliced black olives, ½ cup sliced radishes, and ½ cup chopped fresh parsley or coriander/cilantro.

Jodi's Famous Bean Salad

My daughter Jodi is always asked to bring this terrific bean salad to dinner parties and barbecues. Thank goodness it's so easy to make. My granddaughter Lauren loves it!

19 oz (540 ml) can black beans
19 oz (540 ml) can chickpeas
19 oz (540 ml) can lentils
2 cloves garlic, crushed
1 green and/or red pepper, chopped
1 yellow pepper, chopped
½ cup red onion, chopped
¼ cup coriander/cilantro, minced
¼ cup extra virgin olive oil
¼ cup balsamic vinegar
1 tsp ground cumin (or to taste)
Salt and freshly ground black pepper

1. Rinse beans, chickpeas and lentils; drain well. Combine all ingredients in a large mixing bowl; mix well. Season to taste. Cover and refrigerate. This tastes even better the next day!

Yield: 12 servings. This salad will keep for up to 3 days in the refrigerator if tightly covered.

172 calories per serving, 6.1 g fat (0.7 g saturated), 0 mg cholesterol, 8 g protein, 23 g carbohydrate, 238 mg sodium, 190 mg potassium, 3 mg iron, 8 g fiber, 41 mg calcium

Lauren's Black Bean Salad

My 12-year-old granddaughter Lauren chose her favorite ingredients to create this version of her mother Jodi's bean salad. Lauren adds feta cheese "because I like it!" You can easily substitute chickpeas or kidney beans for the black beans. For more color and fiber, make Tex-Mex Bean Salad.

1 can (19 oz/540 ml) black beans, drained and rinsed
½ cup chopped red onion
2 tbsp extra virgin olive oil
2 tbsp balsamic vinegar
1 tsp minced garlic
Salt and freshly ground black pepper
½ cup crumbled feta cheese

1. Combine the beans, onion, oil, vinegar, garlic, salt, and pepper in a large bowl; mix well. Sprinkle with feta cheese and serve immediately.

Yield: About 3 cups (6 servings of ½ cup each). Recipe can be doubled. Keeps for up to 3 to 4 days in the refrigerator.

131 calories per serving, 14.1 g carbohydrate, 4.2 g fiber, 5 g protein, 7.3 g fat (2.5 g saturated), 11 mg cholesterol, 488 mg sodium, 273 mg potassium, 1 mg iron, 94 mg calcium

Variation
- **Tex-Mex Bean Salad:** Omit feta cheese. Add 1 cup drained corn kernels, 1 red pepper, chopped, and ¼ cup minced fresh cilantro or parsley. Makes about 4 cups. One serving contains 104 calories, 16.8 g carbohydrate, 4.2 g fiber, 4 g protein, 3.6 g fat (0.5 g saturated), and 349 mg sodium.

Lighter Cæsar Salad Dressing

Creamy and delicious. You won't miss the fat!

½ cup nonfat yogurt
¼ cup fat-free or low-fat mayonnaise
1 clove garlic, crushed
¼ cup grated Parmesan cheese
½ tsp Worcestershire sauce
2 tbsp lemon juice (to taste)
¾ tsp salt (to taste)
Freshly ground pepper, to taste

1. Combine all ingredients and mix well; chill. Delicious over romaine lettuce or spinach.

Yield: About 1 cup. Dressing will keep 4 or 5 days in the refrigerator.

15 calories per tbsp, 0.6 g fat (0.4 g saturated), 2 mg cholesterol, 1 g protein, 2 g carbohydrate, 168 mg sodium, 27 mg potassium, 0 mg iron, 0 g fiber, 37 mg calcium

Mediterranean Kidney Bean Salad

This Mediterranean delight is packed with fiber and protein. Serve it with a grain such as bulgur, rice, or quinoa to make it a complete protein dish. This makes a satisfying, nutritious, and delicious salad that's an excellent addition to your lunch box.

1 can (19 oz/540 ml) red or white kidney beans, drained and rinsed
3 green onions, minced
2 cloves garlic (about 2 tsp minced)
½ cup minced fresh parsley
½ red pepper, seeded and chopped
1 cup grape or cherry tomatoes

2 tbsp extra virgin olive oil
2 tbsp lemon juice (preferably fresh)
Salt and freshly ground black pepper
½ tsp dried oregano, basil, thyme, or rosemary, or 1 tbsp minced fresh

1. Combine all the ingredients in a large bowl and toss to mix well. Set aside and let marinate for 10 to 15 minutes before serving.

Yield: 4 servings. Recipe doubles and triples easily. Keeps for up to 3 or 4 days in the refrigerator.

196 calories per serving, 25.4 g carbohydrate, 9.8 g fiber, 8 g protein, 7.7 g fat (1.1 g saturated), 0 mg cholesterol, 446 mg sodium, 561 mg potassium, 3 mg iron, 65 mg calcium

Variations

- **Mediterranean Chickpea Salad:** Substitute chickpeas for kidney beans. Add a handful of pitted black olives and use different-colored peppers such as a combination of red, green, orange, and yellow. Sun-dried tomatoes also make a delicious addition.
- **Mediterranean Bean and Pasta Salad:** Add 2 cups of cooked pasta such as whole-wheat rotini, shells, or macaroni. Don't overcook the pasta: it should be al dente (just cooked but still firm to the bite) to give it a lower glycemic index. Increase the olive oil and lemon juice to 3 tbsp each and use 1 tsp oregano or desired herbs.
- **Mediterranean Mixed Bean Salad:** Double or triple the recipe for a crowd, using a mixture of red or white kidney beans, black beans, and chickpeas. If desired, sprinkle with 1 cup crumbled feta or goat cheese. For an elegant presentation, serve it on a large platter instead of using a salad bowl.

Mixed Greens with Mandarins, Berries and Pears

This scrumptious salad, with its crunchy topping of pistachios, is a perfect pairing of fruits and salad greens. The fat is mainly heart-healthy mono-unsaturated. Your guests will be green with envy when they taste it.

Raspberry Vinaigrette (page 102)
4 cups packed baby spinach or mixed salad greens
1 head romaine lettuce, torn into bite-sized pieces (about 6 cups)
½ cup red onion, thinly sliced
1 can (10 oz/284 ml) mandarin oranges, drained (about 1 cup)
1 cup fresh strawberries and/or raspberries, hulled and halved
½ cup dried cranberries
2 firm ripe pears, peeled, cored, and sliced
2 tsp lemon juice (preferably fresh)
½ cup toasted pistachios or pine nuts, for garnish

1. Prepare the Raspberry Vinaigrette as directed and chill until serving time.
2. Combine the spinach, romaine, onion, oranges, strawberries, and cranberries in a large salad bowl but don't toss. (If desired, the salad can be prepared up to this point several hours in advance and refrigerated.)
3. At serving time, sprinkle the pears with lemon juice to prevent discoloration, and add to the salad. Drizzle the chilled vinaigrette over the salad and toss gently. Garnish with pistachios and serve immediately.

Yield: 8 servings.

221 calories per serving, 25.5 g carbohydrate, 4.4 g fiber, 3 g protein, 13.2 g fat (1.8 g saturated), 0 mg cholesterol, 41 mg sodium, 222 mg potassium, 1 mg iron, 48 mg calcium

Variations
- Instead of pears, use sliced mango or apples. Instead of mandarin oranges, add 1 cup of grapefruit segments. If desired, top the salad with ½ cup crumbled goat cheese just before serving.

Quinoa, Black Bean and Corn Salad

Quinoa (KEEN-wah) has a delicate, nutty flavor and chewy texture. It looks similar to raw sesame seeds. This nutritious salad is a fabulous dish for a buffet and can be expanded into a main course easily. Everyone will be keen on quinoa once they taste this!

2 cups vegetable or chicken broth
1 cup quinoa
1 can (19 oz/540 ml) black beans, drained and rinsed
1 cup corn kernels
1 medium red pepper, seeded and chopped
4 green onions, chopped
¼ cup chopped fresh cilantro or parsley
2 cloves garlic (about 1 tsp minced)
½ tsp ground cumin
¼ to ½ tsp cayenne pepper (or to taste)
3 to 4 tbsp lime or lemon juice (preferably fresh)
3 to 4 tbsp extra virgin olive oil
Salt and freshly ground black pepper

1. Bring the broth to a boil in a medium saucepan over high heat. Place the quinoa in a fine-mesh strainer and rinse under cold running water for 1 to 2 minutes; drain well. (Rinsing removes the bitter coating.)
2. Add quinoa to the boiling liquid. Reduce heat to low and simmer, covered, for 15 minutes. Don't overcook. Remove from heat and let stand, covered, for 5 minutes. Fluff with a fork, transfer to a large bowl and let cool.
3. Add the beans, corn, red pepper, green onions, cilantro, garlic, cumin, and cayenne to the quinoa. Drizzle the lime juice and olive oil over the salad. Season with salt and pepper; toss well. Can be made a day ahead, covered and refrigerated. Adjust seasonings to taste before serving.

Yield: 12 servings of about ¾ cup. Keeps for up to 3 to 4 days in the refrigerator.

137 calories per serving, 21.5 g carbohydrate, 3.9 g fiber, 4 g protein, 4.5 g fat (0.6 g saturated), 0 mg cholesterol, 313 mg sodium, 267 mg potassium, 2 mg iron, 32 mg calcium

Variations

- **Chicken, Spinach and Quinoa Salad:** Arrange a bed of baby spinach leaves on a large platter; top with the quinoa salad. Arrange thinly sliced grilled chicken breasts (warm or cold), roasted red pepper strips, and sliced avocado on top. Pretty delicious!
- **Couscous and Black Bean Salad:** Substitute couscous for quinoa, but reduce broth to 1-½ cups. (No need to rinse or cook the couscous.) Combine the couscous with hot broth in a large bowl, cover and let stand for 10 minutes, until liquid is absorbed. Continue as directed in Step 3.

Chef's Secrets

- *Switch Around:* Quinoa can replace rice or couscous in many recipes and is delicious as a breakfast cereal instead of oatmeal.
- *What's in Store:* Quinoa can be found in natural food stores and many supermarkets. At home, store it in the refrigerator for 3 to 4 months, or freeze for up to 6 months.

Nutrition Notes

- *Go with the Grain:* Quinoa is lower in carbohydrates than most grains and is considered a complete protein because it contains all eight essential amino acids.
- *GI Go!* The glycemic index value for quinoa is 51. It's packed with fiber and is a great source of B vitamins and minerals, including iron, magnesium, phosphorus, and zinc.

Rainbow Tabbouleh Salad

This colorful, vitamin-packed salad is guaranteed to be a winner on any buffet table! This is a wonderful way to use up fresh mint if you grow it in your garden.

⅓ cup bulgur or couscous
⅔ cup boiling water
2 cups minced flat-leaf or curly parsley
1 cup mint leaves
1 green and 1 red pepper
4 firm, ripe tomatoes
4 green onions (scallions)
¼ cup red onion
¼ cup grated carrots
½ English cucumber, seeded and diced
¼–⅓ cup olive oil (to taste)
¼–⅓ cup fresh lemon juice (to taste)
Salt and pepper, to taste
1 tbsp fresh basil, chopped (or 1 tsp dried)
Fresh mint or basil leaves, to garnish

1. In a small bowl, combine bulgur or couscous with boiling water. Let stand for 20 minutes to soften. (Couscous will take only 10 minutes.) Meanwhile, soak parsley and mint in cold salted water for 15 to 20 minutes. Drain and dry well. Trim off tough parsley stems. Remove mint leaves from stems.

2. Mince parsley and mint leaves. Chop vegetables. (Do this in the processor in batches, using on/off turns to retain texture.) Combine parsley, mint, and vegetables in a large mixing bowl. Add drained bulgur or couscous, olive oil, and lemon juice. Mix well. Add salt, pepper and basil. Allow to stand for at least ½ hour for flavors to blend. Garnish with fresh mint or basil leaves.

Yield: 8 servings. Leftovers will keep for 2 or 3 days in the refrigerator.

121 calories per serving, 7.4 g fat (1 g saturated), 0 mg cholesterol, 3 g protein, 14 g carbohydrate, 22 mg sodium, 434 mg potassium, 2 mg iron, 4 g fiber, 47 mg calcium

Variations

- Store bulgur in an airtight container in a cool dark place. It can be stored in the refrigerator for several months, or in the freezer for up to a year.
- Reserve parsley stems and use them when making chicken or vegetable broth.
- Parsley should be well-dried before chopping. Your processor makes quick work of this task. Measure parsley after chopping. You need approximately twice as much before chopping to give you the required amount for this recipe.
- If fresh mint is not available, add 2 teaspoons dried mint. If you don't have dried mint, just leave it out. The salad will still have a delicious, garden-fresh flavor.
- *Variation:* Increase bulgur or couscous to 1 cup for a grain-based tabbouleh. Soak the grain in double the amount of water.
- **Traditional Tabbouleh:** Omit red onion, carrots, cucumber, and basil.
- **Quinoa Tabbouleh:** Use 1 cup of cooked quinoa instead of soaked bulgur or couscous.
- **Greek-Style Tabbouleh:** Crumble or grate ½ cup feta cheese over tabbouleh. Add ⅓ cup sliced black olives. One serving contains 152 calories, 10 g fat (2.5 g saturated) and 98 mg calcium

Raspberry Vinaigrette

If you keep frozen raspberries on hand, you can whip up this fruity dressing in about 30 seconds. It's excellent over grains or greens. For a real taste sensation, drizzle it over grilled asparagus. You'll razzle-dazzle them!

⅓ cup fresh or frozen raspberries (no need to defrost)
⅓ cup extra virgin olive oil
1 tsp Dijon mustard
2 tbsp balsamic vinegar (or 1 tbsp balsamic vinegar and 1 tbsp orange juice)
1 tbsp honey
Salt and freshly ground black pepper

1. In a food processor fitted with the steel blade, process raspberries for 8 to 10 seconds. Add the remaining ingredients and process 10 seconds longer to combine. Transfer to a jar and store in the refrigerator. Shake well before using.

Yield: About ⅔ cup. Recipe doubles and triples easily. Keeps for up to a week to 10 days in the refrigerator.

68 calories per tbsp, 2.5 g carbohydrate, 0.2 g fiber, 0 g protein, 6.5 g fat (0.9 g saturated), 0 mg cholesterol, 12 mg sodium, 4 mg potassium, 0 mg iron, 2 mg calcium

Roasted Sweet Potato Salad

This fiber-filled dish is absolutely addictive. The sweet potatoes become glazed during the roasting process and have a scrumptious candied taste, even though there's only one tablespoon of maple syrup in this recipe. You can double the recipe for a crowd, but if you do, use two baking trays to be sure to spread out the potatoes in a single layer when roasting.

4 medium sweet potatoes, peeled and cut into 1-inch pieces (about 6 cups)
1 red pepper, seeded and cut into 1-inch pieces
2 tbsp balsamic vinegar
4 tsp extra virgin olive oil
1 tsp dried basil
½ tsp salt
¼ tsp freshly ground black pepper

Dressing:
1 tbsp balsamic vinegar
1 tbsp extra virgin olive oil
1 tsp Dijon mustard
1 tbsp pure maple syrup
1 tsp minced garlic
4 green onions, thinly sliced (about ¾ cup)

1. Preheat the oven to 425°F. Line a large baking tray with foil and spray with cooking spray.
2. In a large bowl, combine the sweet potatoes, red pepper, vinegar, oil, basil, salt, and pepper; mix well. Spread out in a single layer on the prepared baking sheet. Bake for 25 to 30 minutes or until golden. Remove from the oven and let cool.
3. Meanwhile, in a large bowl, combine the vinegar, oil, mustard, maple syrup, and garlic. Add the roasted sweet potato mixture and green onions to the dressing; toss to mix well. Serve at room temperature or chilled.

Yield: 8 servings of ½ cup each. Keeps for up to 2 to 3 days in the refrigerator.

126 calories per serving, 20.8 g carbohydrate, 3.1 g fiber, 2 g protein, 4.2 g fat (0.6 g saturated), 0 mg cholesterol, 193 mg sodium, 440 mg potassium, 1 mg iron, 45 mg calcium

Romaine, Avocado and Mango Salad with Citrus Dressing

I love to serve this elegant salad on a large platter—it's perfect for a crowd and pretty as a picture. This tastes best using fresh citrus juices, but use bottled juices if you're in a tight squeeze!

Citrus Dressing:
¼ cup lemon juice (preferably fresh)
¼ cup orange juice (preferably fresh)
½ cup extra virgin olive oil

2 cloves garlic (about 2 tsp minced)

2 tsp Dijon mustard

1 tsp honey

Salt and freshly ground black pepper

Rind of ½ a lemon and ½ an orange (optional)

Salad:

3 large romaine lettuce hearts, trimmed

2 ripe medium avocados, pitted, peeled, and diced

2 mangoes, pitted, peeled, and diced

1 English cucumber, unpeeled, quartered and thinly sliced

½ red onion, thinly sliced (about 1 cup chopped)

½ cup thinly sliced radishes

1 red pepper, seeded and thinly sliced

¼ cup chopped fresh basil or parsley

1 pkg (4 oz/113 g) goat cheese, crumbled

1. Combine the ingredients for the salad dressing in a glass jar, seal tightly, and shake well. Refrigerate until serving time.

2. Wash the romaine leaves well and tear into bite-sized pieces. Dry, in batches, in a lettuce spinner. (Can be prepared up to a day in advance, wrapped in towels and refrigerated.)

3. Arrange the lettuce on a large oval platter. Scatter the avocado, mango, cucumber, onion, and radishes over the lettuce. Top with the red pepper and basil. Just before serving, drizzle the dressing on top and garnish with crumbled goat cheese, if using.

Yield: 16 to 20 servings. Recipe can be halved easily for a smaller crowd.

141 calories per serving, 11.2 g carbohydrate, 3.1 g fiber, 2 g protein, 10.9 g fat (1.5 g saturated), 0 mg cholesterol, 23 mg sodium, 243 mg potassium, 1 mg iron, 33 mg calcium

Variation

- Instead of goat cheese, garnish with 1 cup toasted sliced almonds for a dairy-free calcium boost (and more fiber!).

Chef's Secrets

- *Go for Green!* Other greens, such as baby spinach, arugula, mesclun mix, or Boston lettuce can be added or substituted.
- *Meal Deal:* To turn it into a main dish, top with sliced grilled chicken breasts or poached salmon.

Turkish Eggplant Salad

This sweet and spicy eggplant dish is served in many Middle Eastern restaurants and everyone I know who tries it, loves it. It's absolutely addictive!

1 eggplant (about 1-1/2 lb/750 g)
Salt (for sprinkling on eggplant)
2 tbsp olive oil
2 large onions, chopped
3 cloves garlic (about 1 tbsp minced)
3 cups tomato sauce
2 tbsp lemon juice (preferably fresh)
¼ cup granulated sugar or granular Splenda
Salt and freshly ground black pepper
¼ tsp cayenne pepper
½ tsp cumin
½ tsp dried thyme
2 tbsp minced fresh cilantro or parsley

1. Cut off both ends from the eggplant but don't peel. Cut the eggplant into ½-inch chunks. (You should have about 8 cups.) Place the chunks in a colander and sprinkle with salt to drain out any bitter juices. Let stand for about ½ hour before rinsing and patting dry.

2. Heat oil in a large pot on medium heat. Sauté the onions and garlic for 5 minutes or until softened. Increase the heat to medium high, add the eggplant and sauté for 5 to 7 minutes longer or until softened.

3. Stir in the tomato sauce, lemon juice, sugar, salt, pepper, cayenne, cumin, thyme, and cilantro. Bring to a boil; reduce heat to low and cover partially. Simmer for 25 to 30 minutes, until sauce has thickened, stirring occasionally. Adjust seasonings to taste. When cool, cover and refrigerate. Serve chilled.

Yield: About 6 cups (12 servings of ½ cup each). Keeps 4 or 5 days in the refrigerator. Freezes well for up to 2 months.

75 calories per serving, 13.9 g carbohydrate, 3 g fiber, 2 g protein, 2.4 g fat (0.3 g saturated), 0 mg cholesterol, 322 mg sodium, 150 mg potassium, 1 mg iron, 3 g fiber, 13 mg calcium

Chef's Secrets

- *Appe-Teasers!* This spread makes a delicious addition to any Middle Eastern appetizer platter. Serve it along with Pumpkin Hummus (page 119) or Roasted Eggplant Spread (page 120).
- This also makes a terrific topping for crostini. If desired, sprinkle with low-fat grated mozzarella and broil briefly until the cheese is melted.
- *Using Your Noodle!* Serve hot over pasta as a sauce. For a low-carb version, serve over strands of spaghetti squash instead of pasta.
- *Sweet Choice:* If made with Splenda instead of sugar, one serving contains 61 calories, 10.2 g carbohydrate, and 3 g fiber.

Wheat Berry Salad

This hearty, high fiber salad is based on a recipe that comes from Lee Ann Gallant, a Toronto pediatrician. Lee Ann, a vegetarian, uses organic foods whenever possible to optimize good nutritional health. Use your food processor to speed up the preparation time.

1 cup wheat berries (white or red)
3 cups lightly salted water (for cooking)
1 red pepper, seeded and chopped
4 green onions, thinly sliced
½ cup chopped fresh parsley
½ cup dried cranberries
2 green apples, cored and chopped (don't peel)
½ cup thinly sliced fennel bulb or celery
⅔ cup Raspberry Vinaigrette (page 102)
1 tsp salt
Freshly ground black pepper

1. Place the wheat berries in a colander and rinse with cold water; drain well. Transfer the rinsed wheat berries to a bowl, cover with at least triple the amount of water and soak overnight. Drain well.
2. Combine the wheat berries with lightly salted water in a saucepan and bring to a boil. Reduce heat to low, cover, and simmer for 1 to 1-½ hours or until tender. Drain if necessary and let cool.
3. In a large bowl, combine the wheat berries, red pepper, green onions, parsley, cranberries, apples, and fennel. Add the vinaigrette, salt, and pepper; mix well. Refrigerate for at least 1 hour to blend the flavors.

Yield: 6 cups (12 servings of ½ cup each). Keeps for up to 2 to 3 days in the refrigerator.

162 calories per serving, 24.5 g carbohydrate, 4.1 g fiber, 3 g protein, 6.7 g fat (0.9 g saturated), 0 mg cholesterol, 213 mg sodium, 142 mg potassium, 1 mg iron, 26 mg calcium

Variations

- *Grain Power:* No wheat berries? Use barley, bulgur, couscous, kasha, millet, quinoa, or rice.
- *Herb Magic:* Instead of parsley, use cilantro. Add additional herbs such as basil, oregano, thyme, or rosemary to vary the flavor.

- *Tutti-Fruity:* Instead of dried cranberries, use raisins, dried cherries, dried blueberries, or sliced dried apricots. Instead of apples, use firm plums, peaches, nectarines, or Asian pears.
- *Mix It Up!* Instead of fennel, use jicama, water chestnuts, or hearts of palm.
- *Dress it Up!* Experiment with different salad dressings. Fruity dressings are especially nice.
- *Go Nuts!* Garnish with toasted walnuts, pine nuts, slivered almonds, or pumpkin seeds.

Chef's Secrets

- *Shop Talk!* Wheat berries are available in many supermarkets and health food stores. They come in soft and hard varieties, but this doesn't refer to tenderness. Soft wheat berries are low in gluten and hard wheat berries are high in gluten. Wheat berries will triple in volume when cooked.
- *Chews Right!* Wheat berries have a chewy texture, so be prepared to chew! Choose them to use in salads, as a substitute for rice, pasta, or other grains, or as a breakfast cereal.
- *Mix and Match:* Combine wheat berries with other cooked grains in salads and pilafs. Cooked wheat berries will keep for up to a week in the refrigerator or can be frozen for 3 or 4 months, so cook up a big batch and use them throughout the week in different recipes. Now that's using your grain!

■ SANDWICHES, FILLINGS, DIPS AND SPREADS

If you make your favorite sandwich with high fiber bread, then add fruit or vegetables, you've got a high fiber lunch. (See page 110 for recipes or page 13 for choosing bread at the supermarket.) Try some of the following recipes to boost that fiber content even higher.

For a high fiber, low-calorie snack, dip crudite, or raw vegetables, in one of the scrumptious dips.

Basic Skinny Dip

Use fresh dill for a simply dill-icious dip! Your processor will help you prepare this in a flash.

> ½ cup smooth nonfat cottage cheese
> ½ cup nonfat yogurt
> ¼ cup green onions, minced
> ¼ cup green pepper, minced
> 2 tbsp grated carrots, optional
> 2 tbsp fresh dill, minced (or ½ tsp dried)
> 1 tsp lemon or lime juice
> Salt and pepper, to taste

1. Combine all ingredients and mix well. Chill until serving time. Serve with assorted vegetables.

Yield: About 1-¼ cups. Keeps about 3 or 4 days in the refrigerator.

8 calories per tbsp, 0 g fat (0 g saturated), <1 g cholesterol, 1 g protein, <1 g carbohydrate, 22 mg sodium, 25 mg potassium, 0 mg iron, trace fiber, 15 mg calcium

Chef's Secrets

- If using creamed cottage cheese, drain off excess liquid. Process cottage cheese until completely smooth, about 2 to 3 minutes in the processor. Add remaining ingredients. Blend in with quick on/offs.
- *Skinny Variations:* Use basil instead of dill. Add 1 clove minced garlic, if desired. Substitute ¼ cup minced red pepper or roasted red pepper instead of green pepper. Use minced red onion instead of green onions.

Black Bean Dip

This is skinny dipping at its finest. Serve with Baked Tortilla Chips (page 342) or assorted raw veggies. It's also delicious as a substitute for mayonnaise on wraps and sandwiches.

2 tsp extra virgin olive oil
1 small onion, chopped
2 to 3 cloves garlic, minced
1 can (19 oz/540 ml) black beans, drained and rinsed
⅓ cup water
1 tsp chili powder
¼ tsp cumin
Salt and freshly ground black pepper
2 tsp lemon or lime juice (preferably fresh)
Finely minced fresh cilantro and red pepper, for garnish

1. Heat oil in a large nonstick skillet over medium heat. Add onion and garlic, and sauté for 3 to 4 minutes or until softened. Stir in the black beans, water, chili powder, cumin, salt, and pepper. Simmer uncovered for 5 minutes, stirring occasionally. Stir in lemon juice and remove pan from heat.
2. Using a potato masher, immersion blender, or food processor, mash the bean mixture to the desired consistency.
3. Transfer to a serving bowl, cover, and refrigerate until ready to use. Garnish with cilantro and red pepper and serve chilled.

Yield: About 2 cups. Leftovers keep 3 to 4 days in the refrigerator. Don't freeze.

10 calories per tbsp, 2.0 g carbohydrate, 0.6 g fiber, 0 g protein, 0.2 g fat (0 g saturated), 0 mg cholesterol, 52 mg sodium, 40 mg potassium, 0 mg iron, 5 mg calcium

Chef's Secrets
- *A-Salt with a Deadly Weapon!* To reduce the sodium content of canned beans by half, rinse well. Organic brands are lower in sodium than regular brands but are usually more expensive.
- *Using Your Bean!* The versatile black bean is wonderful in dips, soups, salads, salsas, stews, casseroles, chili, fajitas, and burritos.

Nutrition Note

- Black beans are high in folate, fiber, protein, magnesium, and anti-oxidants. They have a low glycemic index, which helps to stabilize blood sugar levels. Many people find black beans easier to digest than other types of beans.

Ethel Cherry's Smoky Eggplant Dip

This recipe is a winner! The peppers and onions are baked, not fried, in this tasty dish.

2 medium eggplants (about 2 lb/1 kg)
2 green peppers
1 large onion, peeled and sliced
1 clove garlic
1–2 tbsp olive oil
1 tbsp vinegar
½ tsp sugar
1 tsp cumin, or to taste
¼ cup chopped coriander (cilantro) or parsley
4 drops liquid smoke (available in health food or gourmet stores)
Salt and pepper, to taste

1. Preheat oven to 400°F. Place eggplants, peppers, and onions on a sprayed baking sheet and bake until soft. Peppers and onions will take 30 minutes; eggplants will take 45 to 50 minutes.
2. Cut eggplants in half and scoop out flesh. Drain well; discard the skin. Cut peppers in half and discard seeds. Combine all ingredients except eggplant in the processor; chop coarsely. Add eggplant; process with quick on/offs. Transfer to a serving bowl and refrigerate.

Yield: About 4 cups. Serve with toasted pita chips or crackers. Mixture keeps 4 or 5 days in the fridge.

6 calories per tbsp, 0.2 g fat (0 g saturated), 0 mg cholesterol, trace protein, 1 g carbohydrate, <1 mg sodium, 34 mg potassium, trace iron, trace fiber, 2 mg calcium

Garden Vegetable Hummus

This guilt-free hummus can be used as a spread on pita bread or as a filling for tortilla wraps. It's excellent as a dip with veggies, crisp flatbread, or Pita Chips (page 343). Dip "a-weigh" to your heart's delight!

1 can (19 oz/540 ml) chickpeas, drained and rinsed
3 to 4 cloves garlic (about 1 tbsp minced)
½ green pepper, seeded and cut in chunks
½ red pepper, seeded and cut in chunks
4 green onions or 1 medium onion, cut in chunks
¼ cup fresh basil
2 tbsp extra virgin olive oil
2 tbsp lemon juice (preferably fresh)
2 to 3 tbsp tahini (sesame paste)
Salt and freshly ground black pepper
Chopped fresh parsley, for garnish

1. Combine all the ingredients except the parsley in a food processor fitted with the steel blade. Process with quick on/offs to start, then let the motor run until the mixture is very smooth, about 2 minutes, scraping down the sides of the bowl as needed.
2. Transfer the hummus to a serving bowl and sprinkle with parsley. Cover and chill in the refrigerator for 1 to 2 hours before serving. (The hummus will thicken when refrigerated.)

Yield: About 2-½ cups. Keeps about 1 week in the refrigerator. Don't freeze.

21 calories per tbsp, 2.5 g carbohydrate, 0.5 g fiber, 1 g protein, 1 g fat (0.1 g saturated), 0 mg cholesterol, 28 mg sodium, 30 mg potassium, 0 mg iron, 6 mg calcium

Variations

- **Mediterranean Hummus:** Add ½ cup well-drained roasted red pepper and a dash of cumin; blend well. For an Italian twist, substitute pesto for the tahini and cumin.
- **Quick Chickpea Salad:** Instead of puréeing the chickpea mixture in a food processor, combine the drained chickpeas with garlic in a mixing bowl. Omit the tahini. Coarsely chop the peppers and green onions. Add to the chickpeas along with the remaining ingredients and mix well. Chill well. Makes 6 servings of ¾ cup each. One serving contains 150 calories, 21.1 g carbohydrate, 4.4 g fiber, 5 grams protein, and 5.7 g fat (0.8 g saturated).

Healthier Hummus

My original recipe called for ⅔ cup of olive oil and ½ cup of tahini. I reduced the fat considerably and used some of the chickpea liquid to provide moistness. As a shortcut, use canned chickpeas.

> 2 cups cooked chickpeas or 19 oz (540 ml) can chickpeas
> ¼ cup fresh parsley
> 3 cloves garlic
> 1 tbsp olive oil
> 2 tbsp tahini (sesame paste)
> 3 tbsp fresh lemon juice
> Salt and pepper, to taste
> ½ tsp ground cumin
> Dash of cayenne pepper or Tabasco sauce

1. Drain chickpeas, reserving about ½ cup of the liquid. (If using canned chickpeas, rinse under cold running water to remove excess sodium; drain well.)

2. Process parsley and garlic until finely minced, about 15 seconds. Add chickpeas and process until puréed. Add remaining ingredients and process until very smooth, adding enough of reserved chickpea liquid for a creamy texture. Processing time will be about 3 minutes. Chill before serving. Serve as a dip with raw or steamed vegetables, crackers, or toasted pita wedges. Great as a spread on grilled pita bread, focaccia, or bagels.

Yield: About 2 cups. Hummus keeps about 1 week in the refrigerator. Do not freeze.

23 calories per tbsp, 1.1 g fat (0.1 g saturated), 0 mg cholesterol, 1 g protein, 3 g carbohydrate, 1 mg sodium, 34 mg potassium, trace iron, <1 g fiber, 7 mg calcium

Variations

- If desired, omit oil and increase tahini to 3 tablespoons. Although tahini is fairly high in fat, it contains important nutrients such as zinc, iron, and calcium, and provides flavor. Tahini can be found in supermarkets, Middle Eastern groceries, or health food stores.
- To lower the fat in tahini, discard oil that comes to the top of the jar. Less fat, same flavor!
- **Skinnier Hummus:** Omit oil and tahini; add 1 green onion, minced. One serving contains 65 calories and 1 gram of fat.
- **Hummus with Roasted Red Peppers:** Add ½ cup roasted red peppers (homemade or from the jar) to chickpeas. Process until fine. Blend in remaining ingredients until smooth.
- **White or Black Bean Spread:** Instead of chickpeas, substitute white kidney beans or black beans. Instead of the bean liquid, thin the mixture with a couple of spoonfuls of nonfat yogurt.
- For a "handy" light and nutritious meal, spread pita or bagel with any of the variations of Healthier Hummus. Top with sliced tomatoes and cucumber, red onion, red pepper (or roasted pepper strips), and sprouts. Great for the lunch box along with some fresh fruit and a thermos of soup!

Hummus Wraps

Healthier Hummus (previous recipe)
6 flour tortillas or very thin pitas (preferably whole-wheat)
½ cup each of chopped tomato and cucumber
½ cup chopped onions (red or green)
½ cup roasted red peppers, in strips
½ cup alfalfa or bean sprouts

1. Spread ⅓ cup of hummus over each tortilla. Sprinkle tomato, cucumber, and onions over hummus; top with roasted pepper strips and sprouts. Fold bottom of tortilla up about 1 inch, then roll it around filling. Serve immediately, or wrap in plastic wrap and chill overnight.

Yield: 6 servings. (These can be sliced ½-inch thick into pinwheels for the kids' lunch boxes!)

247 calories per serving, 8.8 g fat (0.9 g saturated), 0 mg cholesterol, 9 g protein, 36 g carbohydrate, 239 mg sodium, 313 mg potassium, 3 mg iron, 5 g fiber, 60 mg calcium

Lentil Spinach Paté

The food processor makes quick work out of this easy vegetarian paté. Slices make an excellent vegetarian sandwich filling, or serve hot with tomato sauce as a vegetarian alternative to meat loaf.

10 oz pkg (300 g) frozen chopped spinach
2 medium onions
1 stalk celery
2 cloves garlic, minced
1 tbsp olive or canola oil
3–4 tbsp water (as needed)
19 oz can (540 ml) lentils, rinsed and drained

2 medium carrots, cut into chunks
½ cup fresh parsley
1 cup bread crumbs or matzo meal
½ tsp salt (to taste)
½ tsp pepper
½ tsp each dried basil and dried thyme
2 eggs (or 1 egg plus 2 egg whites)

1. Preheat oven to 350°F. Thaw spinach; squeeze dry. Cut onions and celery in chunks. Process with quick on/offs, until coarsely chopped. Sauté onions, celery, and garlic in oil until golden, about 5 minutes. If veggies begin to stick, add 1 to 2 tablespoons of water. Process lentils, carrots, and parsley until minced, about 20 seconds. Add spinach with remaining ingredients and 2 tablespoons of water. Mix well.
2. Pour mixture into a sprayed 9- by 4-inch loaf pan. Bake uncovered at 350°F for about 45 minutes. A knife inserted into the center of the baked loaf should come out clean. Serve hot or cold.

Yield: 8 to 10 slices. Leftovers will keep for 3 or 4 days in the refrigerator or can be frozen.

177 calories per slice, 4.1 g fat (0.9 g saturated), 53 mg cholesterol, 9 g protein, 27 g carbohydrate, 317 mg sodium, 431 mg potassium, 4 mg iron, 7 g fiber, 105 mg calcium

Tips and Variations

- To serve as an appetizer, let cool 15 minutes. Loosen with a flexible spatula or knife and invert carefully onto a serving plate; chill. Serve with sliced cucumbers, tomatoes, and assorted breads.
- Serve slices topped with tomato sauce. (It's like meat loaf, without the meat!) Perfect with baked potatoes and steamed broccoli.
- **Lentil Burgers:** Prepare mixture as directed in Step 1. In Step 2, heat a little oil in a nonstick skillet. Drop uncooked mixture from a spoon into

skillet. (Use a teaspoon for miniatures, or a large spoon for regular-sized burgers.) Flatten slightly with the back of the spoon. Cook for 3 to 4 minutes on each side, or until golden. Pat with paper towels to remove excess fat. Serve miniatures in mini pitas or regular-sized burgers in hamburger buns. Top with salsa, lettuce, onions, etc. Recipe makes about 3 dozen miniatures or 8 to 10 large burgers.

Pita Empanadas

10 oz pkg (300 g) frozen chopped spinach
4 green onions
1 lb pressed nonfat cottage cheese (or 1 lb 1% low-fat firm tofu)
¼ cup grated Parmesan cheese (or soy cheese)
¼ cup skim milk (or soy milk)
1 tsp dried basil
¾ cup tomato/marinara sauce (bottled or homemade)
Salt and pepper, to taste
6 pita breads (preferably whole-wheat)

1. Pierce spinach package in several places with a sharp knife. Place on a plate and microwave on HIGH for 5 minutes. When cool, squeeze spinach dry. In the processor, mince onions. Add spinach, cheese, milk, and seasonings; process for 20 seconds, until mixed. Preheat oven to 375°F. Split one end of each pita open. Spoon some spinach filling into the open end of each pita, then spoon about 2 tablespoons sauce into each pita. Wrap each pita in foil. Bake at 375°F for 20 minutes, until piping hot.

Yield: 6 servings. Do not freeze.

272 calories per serving, 3.3 g fat (1.1 g saturated), 10 mg cholesterol, 19 g protein, 42 g carbohydrate, 826 mg sodium, 406 mg potassium, 3 mg iron, 3 g fiber, 223 mg calcium

Pumpkin Hummus

They'll never know this scrumptious spread contains pumpkin. The inspiration for this recipe comes from cookbook author and dear friend Kathy Guttman. I added chickpeas to pump up the nutritional profile. It makes a big batch, but you can make half the recipe and use the leftover pumpkin to make Pumpkin Cheesecake (page 308). Keep on pump-in!

6 cloves garlic (about 2 tbsp minced)
¼ cup fresh parsley or cilantro leaves
1 can (19 oz/540 ml) chickpeas, drained and rinsed
¼ cup tahini (sesame paste)
¼ cup lemon juice (preferably fresh)
2 tbsp extra virgin olive oil
1 can (15 oz/425 ml) canned pumpkin (about 2 cups)
2 tsp cumin (or to taste)
1 tsp salt (or to taste)
¼ tsp smoked or Hungarian paprika
¼ tsp cayenne pepper
1 to 2 tsp pure maple syrup (or to taste)
Pumpkin seeds, for garnish

1. In a food processor fitted with the steel blade, process the garlic and parsley until finely minced, about 10 seconds. Add the chickpeas and process until puréed, about 18 to 20 seconds. Add remaining ingredients except the pumpkin seeds and process until very smooth, about 2 minutes. If the mixture is too thick, add a little water.
2. Transfer the puréed pumpkin mixture to a bowl, cover, and refrigerate overnight for maximum flavor. Garnish with pumpkin seeds at serving time.

Yield: About 4 cups. Keeps about 1 week in the refrigerator. Freezes well for up to a month.

19 calories per tbsp, 2.4 g carbohydrate, 0.5 g fiber, 1 g protein, 0.9 g fat (0.1 g saturated), 0 mg cholesterol, 52 mg sodium, 30 mg potassium, 0 mg iron, 6 mg calcium

Chef's Secrets

- *Skinny Dip!* This hummus is delicious as a dip served with raw vegetables or toasted pita wedges. It's also scrumptious as a spread on grilled pita bread and sandwiches.
- *Wrap-ture!* When making wraps, spread tortillas with hummus instead of mayonnaise.
- *Frozen Assets!* Freeze in 1 cup containers. When needed, thaw overnight in the refrigerator and stir before serving.

Roasted Eggplant Spread

This ruby-red spread comes from Penny Krowitz of Toronto, who got it from Melissa Adler. It's absolutely out of this world. I've nicknamed it "Penny's from Heaven!" Serve it on top of salad greens or with wholegrain crackers, flatbread, or toasted pita bread wedges.

1 eggplant (about 2 lb/1 kg), peeled and cut in 2-inch chunks
1 red onion, peeled and cut in 2-inch chunks
2 red peppers, seeded and cut in 2-inch chunks
2 tbsp olive oil
1 tsp salt (or to taste)
¼ tsp freshly ground black pepper
1 whole head garlic (trim and discard the top)
2 tbsp tomato paste

1. Preheat the oven to 400°F. Line a 12- by 18- by 1-inch baking sheet with parchment paper or foil.
2. Combine the eggplant, onion, and peppers in a large bowl. Drizzle with oil and sprinkle with salt and pepper. Mix well. Spread out the vegetables in a single layer on the baking sheet.

3. Drizzle the cut side of the garlic with a few drops of oil, wrap in foil, and place on the baking sheet next to the vegetables.
4. Roast, uncovered and stirring occasionally, at 400°F for 40 to 45 minutes, or until the vegetables are tender but slightly blackened around the edges. Remove from the oven and cool slightly.
5. Transfer the vegetables to a food processor fitted with the steel blade. Squeeze the garlic cloves out of their skins and add to the processor along with the tomato paste. Process, using quick on/off pulses, until coarsely chopped. Transfer to a serving bowl, cover, and refrigerate to allow the flavors to blend.

Yield: About 2-¼ cups. Keeps about 2 weeks in the refrigerator. Freezes well for up to 2 months.

73 calories per ¼ cup, 10.8 g carbohydrate, 3.7 g fiber, 2 g protein, 3.3 g fat (0.5 g saturated), 0 mg cholesterol, 291 mg sodium, 322 mg potassium, 1 mg iron, 25 mg calcium

Roasted Eggplant and Peppers

For a delicious side dish, transfer the roasted vegetables to a serving bowl at the end of Step 4. Don't add the tomato paste or chop the vegetables. Delicious hot or at room temperature.

Chef's Secrets
- *Frozen Assets!* Drop tablespoonfuls of leftover tomato paste onto a parchment paper–lined baking sheet and freeze until solid. Transfer the frozen tomato-paste blobs to a re-sealable plastic bag. Store in the freezer and use as needed: add to soups, stews, and sauces—no need to defrost first.
- *Instant Tomato Sauce!* Another way to use up leftover tomato paste is to mix it with double the amount of water and turn it into tomato sauce.

Rozie's Portobello Mushroom Burgers

Scrumptious! Even non-vegetarians will love these at your next barbecue!

3 tbsp balsamic vinegar
1 tbsp olive oil
Salt and pepper, to taste
4 portobello mushroom caps, 4-inches in diameter
4 slices of Spanish onion
1 cup roasted red peppers (from a jar or homemade), cut in strips
½ cup low-fat grated Mozzarella cheese
¼ cup fresh basil leaves, shredded
4 hamburger buns (or whole-wheat rolls), lightly toasted or grilled

1. Mix together balsamic vinegar, oil, salt, and pepper. Pour over mushroom caps and marinate for 20 to 30 minutes. Preheat grill or broiler. Grill or broil mushroom caps and onion slices about 3 to 5 minutes per side, until nicely browned. Separate onions into rings.
2. To assemble, place a mushroom cap on the bottom of each bun. Arrange onion rings and roasted pepper strips on top of mushrooms. Sprinkle with cheese and basil. Cover with the top of the bun. Wrap in foil and heat on the grill or in a 400°F oven for 5 minutes, until hot.

Yield: 4 servings. Can be made in advance and wrapped in foil. Reheat at serving time.

267 calories per sandwich, 9.2 g fat (3.2 g saturated), 8 mg cholesterol, 12 g protein, 36 g carbohydrate, 517 mg sodium, 374 mg potassium, 4 mg iron, 4 g fiber, 167 mg calcium

Sloppy "Toes"

A calci-yummy vegetarian version of Sloppy Joes, made with spicy tofu cut into toe-shaped strips! This makes a delicious filling for pitas or crêpes, or can be served over rice or polenta as a main dish.

1 lb (500 g) firm tofu
1 large onion, diced
1 red and 1 green pepper, diced
1-½ cups zucchini, diced
4–6 cloves garlic, sliced
2 tsp olive oil
1 tsp Cajun seasoning
½ tsp each dried basil and paprika
1 cup medium salsa (bottled or homemade)
4 hamburger buns (or whole-wheat rolls), halved

1. Place tofu between 2 large plates and weigh it down with a heavy weight (e.g., several large cans). Let stand for 15 minutes to release extra liquid. Drain well. Cut into strips ¾-inch wide by 2-inch long. Preheat oven to 400°F. Spray a 9- by 13-inch casserole with nonstick spray. Combine tofu, onions, peppers, zucchini, and garlic in casserole. Drizzle with olive oil and sprinkle with seasonings. Mix well. Bake uncovered at 400°F for 15 minutes. Turn tofu over and bake 10 minutes longer.
2. Pour salsa over tofu and mix well. Bake 10 minutes longer, until heated through. Heat the buns. Spoon hot mixture over bun halves.

Yield: 8 servings. Reheats well. Do not freeze.

180 calories per serving, 7.4 g fat (1.2 g saturated), 0 mg cholesterol, 12 g protein, 19 g carbohydrate, 273 mg sodium, 351 mg potassium, 7 mg iron, 3 g fiber, 174 mg calcium

Stuffed Pita Pockets

Pita bread makes a perfect holder for these tasty pockets—they're packed with phytonutrients, fiber, and flavor. Pack your pockets with any of the tasty variations for lunch or use miniature pitas for perfect appetizers. It's like eating a salad without the fork!

1 cup Black Bean Dip (page 110)
4 medium whole-wheat pitas
1 cup packed baby spinach leaves or mixed salad greens
½ cup diced green pepper
1 cup diced red pepper
2 plum tomatoes, cored and diced
½ English cucumber, unpeeled and diced
2 green onions, thinly sliced
1 tbsp extra virgin olive oil
1 tbsp lemon juice (preferably fresh)
Salt and freshly ground black pepper
4 tsp roasted sunflower seeds (optional)

1. Prepare the dip as directed. Measure 1 cup and reserve the remainder for another use.
2. Slice each pita open along one edge. Spread the inside of the pita evenly with the dip.
3. Combine the spinach, bell peppers, tomatoes, cucumber, and green onions in a large bowl. Add the olive oil, lemon juice, salt, and pepper; mix well. Spoon some of the vegetable mixture into each pita pocket. Sprinkle with sunflower seeds, if desired.

Yield: 4 servings. Recipe doubles and triples easily. Can be prepared up to 24 hours in advance. Don't freeze.

91 calories per serving, 16.8 g carbohydrate, 3.1 g fiber, 3 g protein, 2.1 g fat (0.3 g saturated), 0 mg cholesterol, 188 mg sodium, 178 mg potassium, 1 mg iron, 18 mg calcium

Variations
- Use White Bean Dip (page 130), Garden Vegetable Hummus (page 113), Pumpkin Hummus (page 119), or Roasted Eggplant Spread (page 120). What a spread!

Stuffed Pita Pockets with Falafel and Tahini

Make Uli's Falafel Enlightened (page 126). Prepare Tahini Sauce (page 287). Make the following accompaniments: shredded lettuce, sliced tomatoes, cucumbers, onions, pickled hot peppers, and pickles. Serve falafel balls in warmed pita pockets. (You need 6 falafel balls for each pita, depending on the size of pitas.) Add desired accompaniments. Drizzle lightly with Tahini Sauce.

319 calories per serving, 6.2 g fat ((0.8 g saturated), trace cholesterol, 12 g protein, 56 g carbohydrate, 1069 mg sodium, 517 mg potassium, 4 mg iron, 6 g fiber, 109 mg calcium

Chef's Secrets
- The pickled hot peppers and pickles provide most of the sodium, so choose your toppings wisely!
- An average pita bread weighs about 2 oz and contains 165 calories, 33 grams of carbohydrate, 0.7 grams of fat, and 1 gram of fiber.
- If you deep-fry the falafel balls instead of baking them, you'll add the equivalent of 1 to 2 tsp fat to your falafel sandwich. Just take a long walk after you indulge so you won't bulge!

Toast Cups

A great low-fat replacement for fatty patty shells! Use very fresh bread for best results.

> 12 slices whole-wheat sandwich bread
> Nonstick spray (olive oil flavor is good)

1. Preheat oven to 350°F. Trim crusts from bread. Spray both sides lightly with nonstick spray. Press each slice into a muffin cup. Bake at 350°F for 12 to 15 minutes, or until golden and crisp.

Yield: 12 toast cups. These can be frozen, but be sure to wrap them airtight to prevent freezer burn!

69 calories per whole-wheat toast cup, 1.2 g fat (0.3 g saturated), 0 mg cholesterol, 3 g protein, 13 g carbohydrate, 148 mg sodium, 71 mg potassium, 1 mg iron, 2 g fiber, 20 mg calcium

> *Suggested Fillings:*
> Black Bean and Corn Casserole (page 291)
> Easy Vegetarian Chili (page 157)
> Simple and Good Ratatouille (page 165)

Uli's Falafel Enlightened

Uli Zamir makes fabulous falafel! He uses the family recipe handed down from his father Shlomo, who sold falafel for 20 years from his kiosk in Kiryat Tiv'on.

> 1 lb (454 g) dried chickpeas (2-¼ cups)
> 8 cups cold water
> 2 slices bread
> ½ bunch fresh parsley (½ cup minced)
> 1 bunch (½ cup minced) coriander/cilantro
> 1 onion, chopped
> 5–6 cloves garlic, minced
> 1 tsp salt

½ tsp pepper, to taste
¾ tsp dried cumin
1 tsp baking soda
4 tsp canola or olive oil

1. Pick over chickpeas and discard any stones or debris. Place in a strainer and rinse thoroughly. Soak in cold water for 24 hours at room temperature (or in the refrigerator if your kitchen is very warm). Drain chickpeas and set aside.

2. Soak bread in a little water but don't squeeze it completely dry. Use a processor or grinder to finely grind chickpeas. (If using the processor, do it in 2 or 3 batches.) Transfer mixture to a large bowl. Grind parsley, coriander, onion, garlic, and bread together until fine. Combine with chickpeas and mix well. Add seasonings, baking soda, and 2 teaspoons of oil. (See note below.) Mixture will be thick. Add a little water (about ⅓ to ½ cup) so that mixture is moist but still holds together.

3. Place oven rack in the lowest position in your oven. Preheat oven to 450°F. Line 2 baking sheets with aluminum foil. Spray lightly with nonstick spray, then brush each one lightly with remaining oil. Shape mixture into 1-inch balls and arrange on baking sheets. Bake uncovered at 450°F for 10 minutes, until bottoms are brown. Carefully turn falafel over. Bake 8 to 10 minutes longer.

Yield: about 6 dozen, depending on size. These reheat well or can be frozen.

27 calories per falafel ball, 0.6 g fat (0.1 g saturated), 0 mg cholesterol, 1 g protein, 4 g carbohydrate, 56 mg sodium, 46 mg potassium, <1 mg iron, 1 g fiber, 9 mg calcium

Note

- Uli does not add oil to the chickpea mixture. Instead, he prefers to deep-fry his falafel in hot oil until crisp and golden. They will float to the surface when done. Drain very well on paper towels.

Vegetable Wraps

This versatile recipe comes from my friend Gloria Guttman, of Toronto. It appears in her heartwarming cookbook, *Cooking Kindness*, which benefits the Israel Cancer Research Fund. Because of the concern with eating raw bean sprouts (uncooked and unwashed sprouts can carry salmonella and E-coli), I've suggested using other greens in this recipe. Overall, these delicious "envelopes" of vegetables and greens deliver healthy, handy meals.

⅓ cup light mayonnaise
2 tsp Dijon mustard
6 large (10-inches) whole-wheat tortillas
1 English cucumber, trimmed and thinly sliced (unpeeled)
1 small red onion, thinly sliced
1 large tomato, finely chopped
1-½ cups packed watercress, baby spinach leaves, or mixed salad greens
1 avocado, peeled, pitted, and thinly sliced
1-½ cups shredded, low-fat mozzarella cheese

1. Mix the mayonnaise with mustard in a small bowl. Lightly spread 1 side of each tortilla with the mayonnaise mixture, leaving ½-inch border around the edges of each tortilla.
2. Place an overlapping row of cucumber slices along the bottom edge of each tortilla, leaving a ½-inch border around the bottom and sides. Place an overlapping row of onion slices on top of the cucumber. Then top with chopped tomato, then watercress, then avocado, ending with cheese. Tightly roll each tortilla: starting from the filling end, roll up partway, fold in both sides, then finish rolling.

Yield: 6 servings. Best served immediately, but can be made a few hours in advance.

403 calories per serving, 40.2 g carbohydrate, 9 g fiber, 14 g protein, 18.0 g fat (5.3 g saturated), 23 mg cholesterol, 724 mg sodium, 349 mg potassium, 1 mg iron, 251 mg calcium

Variations
- *Spread It Around:* Instead of mayonnaise, use Garden Vegetable Hummus (page 113). White Bean Dip (page 130) also makes tasty spreads. Instead of sliced avocado, spread some mashed avocado on these wraps for a heart-healthy spread.
- *Veggie Heaven:* Fill wraps with raw or roasted pepper strips, grated carrots, or green onions. Roasted or grilled vegetables, such as mushrooms, peppers, onions, eggplant, and asparagus also make fantastic additions to a wrap.
- *Go for Protein:* Instead of cheese, fill the wraps with tuna, egg, or salmon salad, or thinly sliced grilled chicken or turkey breast.
- *Dill-icious Delight:* Spread tortillas with light cream cheese. Fill with smoked salmon, sliced cucumbers, onions, and tomatoes. Sprinkle with minced fresh dillweed and roll up.

Vegetarian Harvest Roll-Ups (Fajitas)
Wrap it up! So colorful, so healthy.

2 cups eggplant, unpeeled, cut into strips
1 red and 1 yellow pepper, cut into strips
1 red onion, halved and cut into strips
1 zucchini, unpeeled, cut into strips
2 cups sliced mushrooms
3–4 cloves garlic, crushed
1 tbsp olive oil
2 tbsp balsamic vinegar or lemon juice
Salt and pepper, to taste
2 tbsp minced fresh basil (or 2 tsp dried)
3 soft flour tortillas or very thin pitas (preferably whole-wheat)
½ cup grated low-fat Mozzarella cheese, if desired

1. Either preheat broiler, or preheat oven to 425°F. Mix all ingredients (except tortillas and cheese) together in a large bowl. (May be prepared in advance up to this point, covered and refrigerated for 3 or 4 hours.) Spread in a thin layer on a sprayed foil-lined baking sheet. Place pan on top rack of oven. Either broil for 10 to 12 minutes, or bake uncovered for 25 to 30 minutes, until tender-crisp and golden, stirring once or twice.
2. Spread hot vegetables in a thin layer on tortillas, leaving about 1 inch at the bottom. Sprinkle with cheese. Fold bottom of tortilla up about 1 inch, then roll around filling in a cone shape. Fasten with a toothpick and serve. (To serve these piping hot, heat at 425°F for 3 or 4 minutes.)

Yield: 3 servings. These also reheat well in the microwave. One roll-up takes 45 seconds on HIGH.

289 calories per serving, 8.3 g fat (1.2 g saturated), 0 mg cholesterol, 8 g protein, 49 g carbohydrate, 350 mg sodium, 776 mg potassium, 3 mg iron, 5 g fiber, 47 mg calcium. With cheese, 1 serving contains 337 calories, 11.3 g fat (3.1 g saturated) and 169 mg calcium

White Bean Dip

This quick, versatile mixture is marvelous as a dip with assorted vegetables. Serve with red, green, and yellow pepper strips, sliced cucumbers, baby carrots, and celery sticks. It also makes a super spread on toasted wholegrain or pumpernickel bread.

2 cloves garlic
15 or 19 oz can (425 to 540 ml) white kidney beans (cannellini beans), drained and rinsed
2 tbsp lemon juice (preferably fresh)
2 tbsp extra virgin olive oil
½ tsp cumin
½ tsp salt (or to taste)

¼ tsp freshly ground black pepper

5 to 6 drops hot pepper sauce or ¼ tsp chili powder

Chopped fresh parsley, black olives, and paprika, for garnish

1. Drop the garlic through the feed tube of a food processor fitted with the steel blade while the motor is running. Process until minced, about 10 seconds. Add beans, lemon juice, olive oil, cumin, salt, pepper, and hot pepper sauce. Process until smooth and creamy, about 1 to 2 minutes, scraping down the sides of the bowl as needed. If the mixture is too thick, thin with 2 tbsp water.

2. Transfer the white bean dip to a serving bowl. Cover and chill for 1 to 2 hours before serving. Garnish with parsley, olives, and paprika.

Yield: About 1-½ cups. Keeps about 1 week in the refrigerator in a tightly sealed container. Don't freeze.

19 calories per tbsp, 1.9 g carbohydrate, 0.5 g fiber, 1 g protein, 1 g fat (0.1 g saturated), 0 mg cholesterol, 57 mg sodium, 2 mg potassium, 0 mg iron, 5 mg calcium

Variations

- Prepare as directed, adding ½ cup well-drained roasted red peppers.
- Omit the hot pepper sauce; add 1 tbsp minced fresh dillweed.

■ FISH DISHES

Leftover or canned fish combine well with vegetables to make fine fillings for sandwiches or salads.

Asian Tuna Salad

Try this tasty tuna salad with an Asian twist. It's wonderful in wraps and sandwiches.

½ cup red onion, cut in 1-inch chunks
½ cup seeded red pepper, cut in 1-inch chunks
½ cup celery, cut in 1-inch chunks
1 apple, peeled, cored, and cut in 1-inch chunks
2 cans (6-½ oz/184 g each) water-packed tuna, drained
⅓ to ½ cup light mayonnaise
1 tbsp lemon juice (preferably fresh) or rice vinegar
⅛ tsp wasabi powder
1 tbsp low-sodium soy sauce (optional)

1. In a food processor fitted with the steel blade, combine the onion, bell pepper, celery, and apple; process for about 8 to 10 seconds, until finely chopped.
2. Transfer the mixture to a medium bowl. Add the tuna, mayonnaise, lemon juice, wasabi powder, and soy sauce, if using, and mix well.
3. Cover the bowl and store in the refrigerator until ready to use. Serve chilled.

Yield: 4 servings. Keeps for up to 2 to 3 days in the refrigerator. Don't freeze.

219 calories per serving, 12.4 g carbohydrate, 2 g fiber, 21 g protein, 9.3 g fat (1.7 g saturated), 43 mg cholesterol, 497 mg sodium, 366 mg potassium, 1 mg iron, 28 mg calcium

Variations

- Omit the apple and instead add ½ cup finely chopped jicama or water chestnuts. Instead of wasabi powder, substitute 2 or 3 finely minced radishes.

Creamy Salmon Filling in Toast Cups

This tasty filling can also be used for crêpes.

Toast Cups (page 126)
10 oz pkg (300 g) frozen mixed vegetables
2 tsp butter, margarine, or oil
2 green onions, chopped
1 tbsp flour
1-½ cups skim milk or vegetable broth
1 bay leaf
½ cup grated Parmesan cheese
2 tbsp minced fresh basil (or 1 tsp dried)
Salt and pepper, to taste
2 cans (7-½ oz/213 g) salmon, drained and flaked

1. Prepare Toast Cups. Cook vegetables according to package directions; set aside. In a 4-cup glass measuring cup, microwave butter on HIGH for 30 seconds. Add green onions and microwave for 2 minutes. Stir in flour. Slowly stir in milk (or broth); add bay leaf. Microwave on HIGH for 4 to 4-½ minutes, until bubbling. Stir twice during cooking. Add cheese and seasonings.

2. Combine sauce with salmon and vegetables. (Can be prepared in advance and refrigerated.) Microwave on HIGH for 5 minutes (or 10 minutes if refrigerated), until hot. Adjust seasonings to taste. Discard bay leaf. Serve in Toast Cups.

Yield: 12 pieces (6 large or 12 small servings).

176 calories per piece, 5.8 g fat (2.1 g saturated), 21 mg cholesterol, 14 g protein, 18 g carbohydrate, 450 mg sodium, 307 mg potassium, 2 mg iron, 3 g fiber, 210 mg calcium

Variations

- Serve with a large garden salad. Start off your meal with a big bowl of White Bean Soup (page 184). Fiber-full, flavor-full!
- **Tuna Filling:** Instead of salmon, use 2 cans of water-packed tuna, drained and flaked.

Fast Fish Salad

Fast Fish Salad is a terrific way to use up any leftover cooked fish such as sole, tilapia, whitefish, or salmon. It's delicious as a filling for sandwiches or wraps, on top of salad greens, or as a stuffing for hollowed-out tomatoes or peppers. If you don't have enough fish, add one or two hard-boiled eggs to the mixture.

2 green onions
1 stalk celery
1 small carrot
2 or 3 radishes
2 cups leftover cooked fish (skin and bones removed)
¼–⅓ cup light mayonnaise or Cæsar salad dressing
Salt and freshly ground black pepper

1. In a food processor fitted with the steel blade, process the green onions, celery, carrot, and radishes for 8 to 10 seconds or until minced. Add the fish and mayonnaise. Process with quick on/off pulses, until combined. Season with salt and pepper to taste.
2. Transfer the mixture to a bowl, cover, and store in the refrigerator until ready to use. Serve chilled.

Yield: 4 servings. Recipe easily doubles or triples. Keeps for up to 2 days in the refrigerator. Don't freeze.

138 calories per serving, 4.0 g carbohydrate, 1.0 g fiber, 16 g protein, 6.0 g fat (1.0 g saturated), 45 mg cholesterol, 202 mg sodium, 377 mg potassium, 1 mg iron, 34 mg calcium

Variation

- **Quick Crab Salad:** Substitute 1 lb (500 g) flaked surimi (imitation crab) for cooked fish. Add ½ cup chopped red pepper, 2 tbsp lemon juice, and 4 to 6 drops of hot pepper sauce.

Quick Pickled Salmon

Ready to eat the same day, instead of 4 days! Pat Brody of Winnipeg shared her recipe with my mom.

> 2 lb (1 kg) sockeye or coho salmon, cut into slices (fresh salmon can be used)
> ¾ cup sweet mixed pickles
> ¾ cup pickle juice
> ¾ cup ketchup (low-sodium, if available)
> 1 tbsp mustard seed (or more, to taste)
> 1 tbsp celery seed (or more, to taste)
> 2 tbsp sugar
> 2 tbsp white vinegar
> 1 onion, chopped
> 2 carrots, sliced
> 1 Spanish onion, sliced

1. Rinse fish; drain well. Combine remaining ingredients except Spanish onion and fish in a large pot; bring to a boil. Add fish to hot brine, reduce heat and simmer covered for 7 to 8 minutes. Turn fish over gently and simmer 5 minutes longer.
2. Cool fish slightly, then transfer to a cutting board. Carefully remove skin and center bone. Place Spanish onion slices in an oblong casserole. Put fish on top and cover with brine. When completely cool, cover and refrigerate.

Yield: 6 servings. Delicious hot or cold. Fish keeps a week in the refrigerator or may be frozen.

354 calories per serving, 12.7 g fat (2.2 g saturated), 91 mg cholesterol, 31 g protein, 29 g carbohydrate, 463 mg sodium, 747 mg potassium, 2 mg iron, 3 g fiber, 87 mg calcium

Chef's Secret

- Pickles, pickle juice, and ketchup are high in sodium. Pickle juice is not included in the nutritional analysis; it is used just for marinating the salmon but is not eaten.

Tuna Caponata

This is similar to ratatouille, but includes tuna, capers, and raisins. Vinegar and brown sugar give this versatile vegetarian dish a lovely sweet and sour flavor.

2 lb (1 kg) eggplant, unpeeled
Salt, to taste
1 tbsp olive oil
2 medium onions, chopped
2 stalks celery, chopped
1 red pepper, chopped
3 cloves garlic, minced
3 cups mild salsa or tomato sauce
3 tbsp balsamic or red wine vinegar
1 tbsp brown sugar or maple syrup
Freshly ground pepper, to taste
1 bay leaf
¼ cup raisins
3 tbsp capers
½ cup pitted sliced black olives
6-½ oz can (184 g) water-packed tuna, drained and flaked

1. Cut eggplant into 1-inch pieces. Put into a colander and sprinkle with salt. Place a plate on top of eggplant and top with several cans. Let stand for 30 minutes. Rinse thoroughly. Pat dry with towels.

2. Spray a large, heavy-bottomed pot with nonstick spray. Add oil and heat on medium-high heat. Sauté onions, celery, and red pepper for 5 minutes. Add garlic and eggplant. Sauté a few minutes longer, stirring occasionally. If necessary, add a little water to prevent sticking.

3. Add remaining ingredients except olives and tuna. Bring to a boil, reduce heat and simmer covered for 25 to 30 minutes, stirring occasionally. Remove from heat and let cool. Stir in olives and tuna. Adjust seasonings to taste. Discard bay leaf. Refrigerate overnight to allow flavors to blend.

Yield: 8 to 10 servings. Keeps about 10 days in the refrigerator, or can be frozen if you omit tuna. Add tuna after Caponata has defrosted.

143 calories per serving, 3.3 g fat (0.5 g saturated), 7 mg cholesterol, 9 g protein, 22 g carbohydrate, 531 mg sodium, 615 mg potassium, 2 mg iron, 6 g fiber, 80 mg

Chef's Serving Suggestions!

- Serve chilled in Toast Cups (page 126), or place a scoop on a large, fresh leaf of Boston lettuce. Garnish with tomato and cucumber slices. Perfect with Honey Mustard Carrot Salad (page 191).
- **Stuffed Pasta Shells:** Use Caponata as a stuffing for cooked jumbo pasta shells. Top with tomato sauce and sprinkle lightly with grated low-fat mozzarella cheese. Bake uncovered at 350°F for 20 minutes, until bubbling hot.
- Serve with Black Bean Soup (page 73).
- Caponata makes an excellent vegetable side dish if you omit the tuna. It can also be served as a dip or spread with Pita or Baked Tortilla Chips (page 342), crackers, or assorted breads.

■ CHICKEN AND TURKEY

Like all animal protein, poultry has no fiber, but it performs well in a variety of high fiber salads and stir-fry dishes.

Asian Chicken and Noodle Salad

This aromatic Asian salad is a favorite of Judy Gruen of Los Angeles, author of *Till We Eat Again: Confessions of a Diet Dropout.* Thank goodness laughing burns calories—I lost three pounds reading about her weight-loss adventures!

Asian Dressing:
3 tbsp low-sodium soy sauce
3 tbsp rice vinegar
2 tbsp Asian (toasted) sesame oil
2 tbsp canola oil
1 tbsp minced fresh ginger
2 cloves garlic (about 2 tsp minced)
½ tsp granulated sugar
¼ tsp freshly ground black pepper
¼ tsp Chinese five-spice powder

Noodle Salad:
2 cups cooked slivered chicken breasts
1 pkg (16 oz/500 g) soba noodles, cooked (or substitute your favorite whole-wheat pasta)
1 cup sliced celery
2 cups bean sprouts
½ cup sliced green onions
¼ lb (125 g/2 cups) snow peas, blanched for 1 minute, then sliced diagonally into 1-inch pieces
1 to 2 tbsp toasted sesame seeds
3 cups baby spinach or mixed salad greens, well-packed

1. *Dressing:* Combine all ingredients for the dressing in a large bowl and mix well. (Can be made in advance; it will keep for 1 to 2 weeks in the refrigerator in a tightly closed container.)
2. Add the cooked chicken to the dressing and let marinate at least 30 minutes. Add all the other salad ingredients except for the spinach and toss to combine. Refrigerate until serving time. Add the spinach and toss to combine.

Yield: 6 servings as a main dish.

483 calories per serving, 68.4 g carbohydrate, 5.4 g fiber, 32 g protein, 12.2 g fat (1.7 g saturated), 40 mg cholesterol, 510 mg sodium, 411 mg potassium, 4 mg iron, 74 mg calcium

Chef's Secrets

*   *Get Dressed!* This Asian dressing is also delicious on coleslaw, salad greens, pasta, or couscous. One tbsp contains 49 calories, 0.9 g carbohydrate, 0.1 g fiber, and 5.1 g fat (0.5 g saturated).
*   *Spice It Up!* Chinese five-spice powder consists of equal parts of cinnamon, cloves, fennel seed, star anise, and Szechuan peppercorns. It adds fabulous flavor to almost any Asian dish. You can find it in Asian markets and most supermarkets.
*   *Pass the Buck-Wheat!* Soba are spaghetti-shaped noodles made from buckwheat flour and wheat flour. These Japanese noodles, available in health food stores, are brownish-grey and cook in 5 minutes. They are an excellent whole-grain alternative to refined wheat flour noodles or pasta.
*   *Using Your Noodle!* Adding chicken and vegetables to pasta dishes lowers the glycemic index. To lower the carbs and GI value, use double the amount of chicken, half the amount of noodles and add more vegetables. Judy often adds diced red pepper, jicama, and baby corn for color and flavor.
*   *Squash, Anyone?* You can cut the carbs by two-thirds if you substitute cooked spaghetti squash for the noodles. Refer to Spaghetti Squash with Roasted Vegetables (page 295) for cooking method. One serving of salad will contain 265 calories, 22.6 g carbohydrate, 5.5 g fiber, and 19 g protein.

Chicken Mango Salad with Peanut Dressing

I've transformed my recipe for Peanut Sauce into a sensational salad dressing by adding fruit juice to thin it down. You'll go nuts when you try it! Roasted or grilled chicken turns this into a main dish salad. How "chick" is that?

Peanut Dressing:
Peanut Sauce (page 283)
¼ cup pineapple, mango, or freshly squeezed orange juice

Salad:
1 pkg (10 oz/300 g) mixed salad greens
1 red pepper, cut in strips
4 green onions, sliced on the diagonal
1 cup snow peas, ends trimmed
1 can (8 oz/227 g) sliced water chestnuts, drained
4 roasted or grilled boneless, skinless single chicken breasts, thinly sliced
1 mango, peeled, pitted, and diced
Chopped peanuts, for garnish

1. In a small bowl, combine the peanut sauce with juice and mix well. Reserve ½ cup dressing to drizzle over the salad. Cover and refrigerate the remaining dressing for another time.
2. In a large bowl, combine the salad greens, red pepper, onions, snow peas, and water chestnuts. (Dressing and salad mixture can be prepared in advance and refrigerated separately.)
3. At serving time, transfer the salad mixture to a serving platter. Arrange the chicken slices and mango on top. Drizzle with reserved dressing and garnish with chopped peanuts.

Yield: 4 servings as a main dish. Recipe doubles and triples easily.

330 calories per serving, 31.7 g carbohydrate, 6.4 g fiber, 34 g protein, 7.9 g fat (1.7 g saturated), 73 mg cholesterol, 456 mg sodium, 816 mg potassium, 4 mg iron, 98 mg calcium

Curried Chicken, Red Pepper and Mango Salad

This salad is so pretty and it's packed with potassium! Some people are sensitive to mangoes and may develop a red, itchy rash when peeling them. If this applies to you, just wear rubber gloves!

4 cooked skinless chicken breasts, cut in strips
6 cups mixed salad greens
1 mango, peeled
2 red peppers, halved and thinly sliced
1 cup red onion, thinly sliced
½ cup grated carrots
12 cherry tomatoes, halved
2 tbsp balsamic or rice vinegar
1-½ tbsp olive oil
½ tbsp sesame oil
2 tbsp orange juice
1 tbsp honey
1 clove garlic, minced
Salt and pepper, to taste
2 tbsp toasted slivered almonds, optional

1. Prepare chicken salad (or chicken) as directed. Wash and dry salad greens; arrange on individual plates. Place chicken on greens. Slice mango from the outside through to the middle, saving any juices. Cut away the pit. Arrange sliced mangoes attractively around edge of plate. Garnish with sliced peppers, red onion, carrots, and tomatoes. Cover and refrigerate until serving time.

2. Blend vinegar, olive and sesame oils, orange juice, reserved mango juice, honey, and garlic. Season with salt and pepper. Drizzle over salad just before serving. Sprinkle with nuts.

Yield: 6 servings.

276 calories per serving, 8 g fat (1.5 g saturated), 64 mg cholesterol, 26 g protein, 26 g carbohydrate, 189 mg sodium, 753 mg potassium, 2 mg iron, 5 g fiber, 75 mg calcium

Rozie's Freeze with Ease Turkey Chili

3 onions, chopped
2 tbsp olive oil, divided
2 cups peppers, chopped (use a mixture of red, green, and yellow peppers)
2 cups sliced mushrooms
3–4 cloves garlic, crushed
3 lb minced turkey (preferably turkey breast)
19 oz (540 ml) can red kidney beans
19 oz (540 ml) can white beans
28 oz can (796 ml) puréed Italian tomatoes
3 cups tomato sauce
2 cans (5-½ oz/156 ml) tomato paste
19 oz (540 ml) can tomato juice
Salt and pepper, to taste
2 tbsp chili powder (or to taste)
1 tsp each basil and oregano (or to taste)

1. Spray a large pot with nonstick spray. Heat 1 tablespoon oil on medium heat. Add onions and sauté for 5 to 7 minutes. Add peppers and mushrooms; sauté 5 minutes longer, until tender. Add a little water if veggies begin to stick or burn. Remove veggies from pot and set aside. Heat remaining oil. Add turkey and brown on medium high heat, stirring often. Rinse and drain beans. Add with remaining ingredients to pot. Simmer uncovered for 1 hour, stirring occasionally. Adjust seasonings to taste.

Yield: 15 servings. Reheats and/or freezes well. Freeze in meal-sized batches. Serve over pasta or rice.

285 calories per serving, 3.3 g fat (0.6 g saturated), 66 mg cholesterol, 32 g protein, 34 g carbohydrate, 474 mg sodium, 1164 mg potassium, 4 mg iron, 9 g fiber, 68 mg calcium

Chef's Secret
- If using cooked turkey, add to chili during last 15 minutes of cooking.

Tuscan Grilled Chicken Salad

This scrumptious meal-in-one salad is packed with vitamins, minerals, and phytonutrients. If you don't like rosemary, substitute other dried or fresh herbs such as oregano, basil, or thyme. This dish multiplies easily and can be prepared in advance, so it's ideal for entertaining.

Dressing:
½ cup extra virgin olive oil
3 tbsp balsamic vinegar
3 cloves garlic, minced
1 tbsp minced fresh rosemary (or 1 tsp dried rosemary)
½ tsp salt
Freshly ground black pepper

Salad:
6 skinless, boneless, single chicken breasts
3 red peppers, cut in quarters
6 large portobello mushrooms, stems discarded
1 pkg (10 oz/300 g) fresh baby spinach or mixed salad greens
1 medium red onion, quartered and thinly sliced
Salt and freshly ground black pepper
¼–⅓ cup toasted sliced almonds, for garnish

1. *Dressing:* In a small bowl, whisk together oil, vinegar, garlic, rosemary, salt, and pepper.

143

2. Place chicken breasts in a re-sealable plastic bag and add ¼ cup of the dressing. (Reserve remaining dressing.) Marinate chicken for at least 30 minutes or up to 48 hours in the refrigerator. Turn bag over occasionally to coat chicken on all sides.

3. Preheat grill. Brush peppers and mushrooms with 3 tbsp of reserved dressing. Grill them over indirect medium-high heat, turning once, about 8 to 10 minutes. Grill chicken breasts over indirect heat until juices run clear and meat is no longer pink in the center, about 8 to 10 minutes (4 to 5 minutes per side). Discard any leftover marinade from the chicken.

4. Remove chicken, peppers, and mushrooms from the grill and transfer them to a cutting board. Cut into ½-inch wide strips. (Can be prepared up to a day in advance and refrigerated until serving time.)

5. At serving time, combine the spinach and onion in a large bowl. Drizzle with reserved salad dressing and toss well. Season with salt and pepper. Transfer spinach mixture to a large serving platter or individual serving plates. Add the grilled peppers and mushrooms. Top with sliced chicken and sprinkle with almonds.

Yield: 6 servings as a main dish.

405 calories per serving, 15.9 g carbohydrate, 5 g fiber, 31 g protein, 24.0 g fat (3.2 g saturated), 73 mg cholesterol, 342 mg sodium, 770 mg potassium, 3 mg iron, 77 mg calcium

Chef's Secret

- *Save Time, Save Calories!* Replace marinade with ⅔ cup commercial low-calorie balsamic or Italian vinaigrette. One serving contains 247 calories and 6.6 g fat (1.2 g saturated).

■ PASTA DISHES

If you stick with whole-wheat, pasta's always a high fiber meal, no matter the sauce.

Broccoli Pasta Quickie

Broccoli, Mushroom and Pepper Sauté (page 201)
3 cups cooked pasta (e.g., ruffles, rotini, or shells)

1. Toss broccoli mixture together with pasta and serve immediately. Makes 4 to 6 servings.

202 calories per serving, 3.4 g fat (0.5 g saturated), 0 mg cholesterol, 8 g protein, 36 g carbohydrate, 23 mg sodium, 400 mg potassium, 3 mg iron, 4 g fiber, 51 mg calcium

Fasta Pasta

This is a great last-minute dish to make when you're rushed for time.

2 cups rotini or macaroni
1 onion, chopped
2 tsp canola oil
1 lb extra-lean ground turkey, chicken, or beef
2-½ cups bottled marinara/spaghetti sauce
½ cup water
3 cups frozen mixed vegetables
Salt, pepper, and garlic powder, to taste

1. Cook pasta in boiling salted water according to package directions. Drain and rinse; set aside. Meanwhile, spray a large pot with nonstick spray. Sauté onion briefly in oil. Add meat and brown for 6 to 8 minutes, stirring often. Remove excess fat from browned meat mixture by placing it in a fine strainer and rinsing it quickly under running water. Return meat to pan along with tomato sauce, water, and frozen vegetables. Cover and simmer for 15 minutes, stirring occasionally. Stir in pasta and cook 5 minutes longer, until heated through. Season to taste.

Yield: 6 servings. Leftovers will keep for a day or 2 in the refrigerator or can be frozen.

357 calories per serving, 7 g fat (0.9 g saturated), 55 mg cholesterol, 28 g protein, 48 g carbohydrate, 615 mg sodium, 877 mg potassium, 4 mg iron, 8 g fiber, 68 mg calcium

Hi-Fiber Vegetarian Lasagna

For smaller families, make several smaller lasagnas in loaf pans and freeze them. So handy!

> 4 cups High-Fiber Vegetarian Pasta Sauce (page 271) (or Cheater's Hi-Fiber Pasta Sauce, page 270)
> 9 lasagna noodles, cooked, drained and laid flat on towels
> 2 cups low-fat ricotta or dry cottage cheese
> 1-½ to 2 cups grated low-fat mozzarella cheese
> 6 tbsp grated Parmesan cheese

1. Place about ⅓ of the sauce in the bottom of a lightly greased or sprayed 9- by 13-inch casserole. Arrange 3 lasagna noodles in a single layer over sauce. Top with half of the ricotta, ⅓ of the mozzarella, and half of the Parmesan. Repeat with sauce, noodles and cheese. Top with noodles, sauce and mozzarella cheese. (Can be made in advance up to this point and refrigerated or frozen. Thaw before cooking.) Bake uncovered in a preheated 375°F oven for 40 to 45 minutes. Let stand for 10 to 15 minutes for easier cutting.

Yield: 10 to 12 servings. Freezes and/or reheats well.

271 calories per serving, 9.3 g fat (5.2 g saturated), 27 mg cholesterol, 18 g protein, 30 g carbohydrate, 239 mg sodium, 408 mg potassium, 2 mg iron, 5 g fiber, 328 mg calcium

Chef's Secrets
- Fresh lasagna noodles or no-cook packaged noodles can be used. No need to precook them!
- Dry cottage cheese is more difficult to spread than ricotta, so thin it with a few drops of skim milk. If using creamed cottage cheese, purée it in the processor for 2 to 3 minutes, until smooth.
- Don't fuss too much about spreading the cheese evenly. Drop it by spoonfuls over the noodles. Don't worry if there are any spaces. The cheese will spread during baking.
- *Variation:* Instead of ricotta cheese, substitute So-Low Alfredo Sauce (page 286).

Many Color Vegetable Lasagna
(See recipe, page 273)

Mexican Pasta with Beans
Full of fiber, full of beans, full of flavor!

2-7-18

OK

not great

2 tsp olive oil
1 onion, chopped
2 cloves garlic, crushed
1 green or red pepper, chopped
1 jalapeño or chili pepper, seeded and minced
19 oz can (540 ml) can kidney or black beans, rinsed and drained
28 oz can (796 ml) diced tomatoes
Salt and pepper, to taste
½ tsp oregano
1 lb spaghetti, penne, or rotini
¼ cup chopped coriander (cilantro)
¼ cup chopped green onions, to garnish
Grated low-fat cheddar cheese, optional

1.   Heat oil in a nonstick skillet. Sauté onion, garlic, and peppers for 5 minutes. Add beans, tomatoes, salt, pepper, and oregano. Simmer uncovered for 10 to 15 minutes, stirring occasionally. Meanwhile, cook pasta according to package directions. Drain well but do not rinse, reserving ½ to ¾ cup of the cooking water. Mix pasta with sauce and reserved cooking water. Serve on hot plates. Garnish with coriander and green onions. If desired, sprinkle lightly with grated cheese.

Yield: 6 servings. Sauce can be frozen.

456 calories per serving, 2.4 g fat (0.3 g saturated), 0 mg cholesterol, 24 g protein, 83 g carbohydrate, 12 mg sodium, 149 mg potassium, 2 mg iron, 12 g fiber, 31 mg calcium

Chef's Secret

- Wear rubber gloves or put plastic bags on your hands when handling hot peppers. The smaller the pepper, the hotter it is. Don't rub your eyes or touch sensitive body parts after handling peppers.

Pasta Primavera

This scrumptious, vegetable-packed dish is also packed with nutrients, including calcium, folate, and fiber. Use this recipe as a springboard for your favorite vegetables. Spring forward to good health!

1 pkg (12 oz/375 g) whole-wheat pasta (such as rotini, penne, bow ties, or macaroni)
2 tbsp olive oil
1 red onion, halved and thinly sliced
1 red pepper, halved, seeded, and thinly sliced
3 cloves garlic (about 1 tbsp minced)
1 medium zucchini, halved and thinly sliced
1 pound (500 g) thin asparagus, trimmed and cut in 1-inch pieces
6 plum tomatoes, coarsely chopped
2 tsp salt (or to taste)

¼ tsp freshly ground black pepper

4 cups lightly packed fresh baby spinach

½ cup fresh chopped basil

6 tbsp grated Parmesan cheese

1. Bring a large pot of salted water to a boil 15 to 20 minutes before cooking the pasta.

2. Meanwhile, heat the oil in a large nonstick wok or deep skillet over medium. Add the onion, pepper, and garlic; sauté for 3 to 4 minutes or until tender-crisp. Add the zucchini, asparagus, and tomatoes, and mix well. Stir in the salt and pepper.

3. Reduce heat to low and simmer, uncovered, for 10 to 15 minutes, stirring occasionally. Stir in the spinach and fresh basil, and cook for 2 minutes longer. (If desired, the sauce can be prepared up to a day in advance and refrigerated overnight. Reheat it just before serving.)

4. While the sauce is simmering, cook the pasta in boiling water according to package directions or until al dente. Ladle out about ½ cup of cooking liquid and set aside. Drain the pasta.

5. Stir ⅓ to ½ cup of the reserved cooking liquid into the sauce. Divide the pasta among 6 bowls and top with the sauce. Sprinkle with cheese and serve immediately.

Yield: 6 servings. Keeps for up to 2 days in the refrigerator. Reheats well in the microwave. Don't freeze.

350 calories per serving, 59.1 g carbohydrate, 9.5 g fiber, 13 g protein, 8 g fat (1.6 g saturated), 4 mg cholesterol, 516 mg sodium, 699 mg potassium, 3 mg iron, 129 mg calcium

Variations

- Add 2 cups sliced mushrooms to the onions and bell peppers; use yellow, orange, or purple bell peppers as well as red.
- Instead of asparagus, use green beans or snow peas. Sun-dried tomatoes and/or roasted red peppers also make a tasty addition.

- Use 1 tsp each of dried oregano and thyme instead of basil, or substitute Italian seasoning.
- Instead of Parmesan cheese, top the pasta with ½ to 1 cup crumbled goat cheese or grated low-fat mozzarella cheese.
- Omit the Parmesan cheese. Add an 8 oz (250 g) package of smoked salmon, coarsely chopped, along with the spinach. Imitation flaked crabmeat is also an excellent option.

Penne Pesto with Tuna and Veggies

Presto—penne pesto! This versatile pasta dish is perfect when you're rushed for time. Pasta and veggies are cooked in the same pot and then the pot is used to combine all the ingredients, saving on clean-up.

1 pkg (16 oz/500 g) penne pasta (preferably whole-wheat)
3 cups frozen mixed vegetables
⅓ cup Best-O Pesto (page 282) or store-bought pesto
2 cans (6 oz/170 g each) flaked, water-packed tuna, well-drained
Salt and freshly ground black pepper
1 cup grated low-fat mozzarella cheese

1. Preheat the oven to 375°F. Spray a 9- by 13-inch glass baking dish with cooking spray.
2. Bring a large pot of salted water to a boil. Add the pasta and cook for 7 to 8 minutes. Add the frozen vegetables and cook for 2 to 3 minutes longer or until the pasta is al dente.
3. Drain the pasta and vegetables and return to the pot. Stir in the pesto, tuna, salt, and pepper; mix well.
4. Spread the pasta-tuna mixture evenly in the prepared baking dish. Sprinkle evenly with cheese. (If desired, the dish can be prepared up to this point and refrigerated up to 24 hours.)
5. Bake, uncovered, for 20 to 25 minutes or until golden and piping hot.

Yield: 8 servings. Keeps for up to 2 to 3 days in the refrigerator; reheats well. Freezes well for up to 2 months.

384 calories per serving, 46.2 g carbohydrate, 6.4 g fiber, 32 g protein, 7.4 g fat (2.0 g saturated), 33 mg cholesterol, 412 mg sodium, 495 mg potassium, 3 mg iron, 156 mg calcium

Variations

- *Using Your Noodle:* Try different shapes and colors of pasta, such as rotini, macaroni, or bow ties and different combinations of frozen mixed vegetables such as broccoli, cauliflower, green beans, carrots, or green peas.
- *Switch to Salmon:* Although one can (6 oz/170 g) of drained tuna measures about ⅔ cup and one can (7-½ oz/213 g) of drained salmon measures about 1 cup, using salmon instead of tuna won't affect the recipe.
- *Using Your Bean:* Instead of tuna or salmon, add 1 can (19 oz/540ml) kidney beans, drained and rinsed. Omit the cheese, if you want to lower the calorie, sodium, and fat content.
- *The Choice Is Yours:* Store-bought pesto is convenient but is higher in calories, fat, and sodium. Try Besto-O Pesto (page 282) in this recipe.

Chef's Secret

- *Frozen Assets:* Instead of a large baking dish, divide the mixture and spread evenly in individual foil containers that have been sprayed with cooking spray. Sprinkle with cheese. Wrap well and freeze for a future meal. There's no need to thaw before using; just bake, covered, for 15 minutes, then uncover and bake for 10 minutes more or until piping hot.

Nutrition Notes

- *GI Go!* Pasta has a lower glycemic index than bread because the starch is in a denser form and is digested more slowly. If pasta is cooked al dente, it has an even lower glycemic index. "Al dente" means that pasta is just cooked but still firm, not too soft or overcooked.
- *Turn Up the Volume:* By adding vegetables and tuna to the pasta, you increase the portion size and lower the glycemic index.

1-7-18   Good

Penne with Roasted Peppers and Sun-Dried Tomatoes

The tomato sauce is used to moisten the pasta and give it a hint of color.

1 pkg (1 lb/500 g) penne or other pasta
1 cup jarred roasted red peppers, cut in strips
½ cup sun-dried tomatoes
2 medium onions, chopped (or cut in strips)
1 tbsp olive oil
1 zucchini, sliced (optional)
3 cloves garlic, minced
⅓ cup fresh basil, finely chopped
¼ cup grated Parmesan cheese
1-½–2 cups tomato sauce
Salt and pepper, to taste

1. Set a large pot of water up to boil for the pasta. Meanwhile, cut jarred peppers into strips. Soak sun-dried tomatoes in boiling water for 10 to 15 minutes, until rehydrated. Drain and dry well; cut into strips.
2. Sauté onions in olive oil on medium heat for 3 to 4 minutes. Add zucchini and garlic; cook 3 to 4 minutes longer. If necessary, add a little water to prevent burning. Cook pasta in boiling salted water for 10 to 12 minutes, until al dente. Drain well. Combine all ingredients and mix well. Delicious hot or at room temperature.

Yield: 6 servings. Reheats and freezes well. If necessary, add a little extra tomato sauce when reheating.

343 calories per serving, 5.2 g fat (1.4 g saturated), 3 mg cholesterol, 13 g protein, 62 g carbohydrate, 683 mg sodium, 509 mg potassium, 4 mg iron, 5 g fiber, 100 mg calcium

Chef's Secrets

- If using roasted peppers from the jar, drain and rinse them thoroughly to remove excess sodium.
- *Chef's Short-Cut!* Instead of soaking the sun-dried tomatoes, add them along with the pasta to the boiling water. They will rehydrate by the time the pasta has cooked!
- **Pasta with Mushrooms, Roasted Peppers and Sun-Dried Tomatoes:** Soak ¼ to ⅓ cup of dried exotic mushrooms (e.g., porcini, shiitake) in boiling water to cover. (Soak them separately from the sun-dried tomatoes. The soaking liquid from mushrooms can be added to your favorite vegetable broth to enhance the flavor.) Add drained mushrooms to the onions along with zucchini and garlic; sauté for 3 or 4 minutes.
- **Pasta with Pesto:** Omit tomato sauce and Parmesan cheese. Add Pesto Alfredo Sauce (page 287) to pasta mixture. This is lovely with bow tie pasta.

Pesto Pasta Salad

Excellent for a summer salad buffet, and so pretty. If you don't have pesto on hand, add 2 cloves of freshly crushed garlic and 3 tablespoons grated Parmesan cheese.

12 oz pkg (340 g) spiral pasta or 3-color rotini
2 cups frozen mixed vegetables (e.g., broccoli, cauliflower, and carrots)
6 green onions, chopped
2 green peppers, chopped
1 red pepper, chopped
¼ cup parsley, minced
¼ cup fresh basil leaves, minced
3 tbsp Best-O Pesto (page 282), to taste
3 tbsp extra virgin olive oil
2 tbsp lemon juice
⅓–½ cup nonfat yogurt or mayonnaise
Salt and pepper, to taste

1. Cook pasta according to package directions. Drain well. Cook vegetables according to package directions. Let cool. In a large bowl, combine all ingredients and mix well. Adjust seasonings to taste. Chill at least 2 or 3 hours or overnight to allow flavors to blend.

Yield: 10 servings. Leftovers will keep for 2 or 3 days in the refrigerator. Do not freeze.

209 calories per serving, 5.7 g fat (0.8 g saturated), trace cholesterol, 7 g protein, 34 g carbohydrate, 35 mg sodium, 256 mg potassium, 2 mg iron, 4 grams fiber, 59 mg calcium

Variations

- Substitute bow tie pasta for 3-color pasta. As a vegetarian main dish, add 1 to 2 cups canned chickpeas, rinsed and drained. If needed, add a little extra yogurt or mayonnaise to moisten.
- **Pareve Pasta Salad:** Use low-fat mayo instead of yogurt. Omit pesto; add 1 teaspoon Dijon mustard.
- **Salmon Pasta Salad:** Add 2 cups of cooked/canned salmon, in chunks. Dill can replace basil.

■ VEGETARIAN DISHES

Vegetarian cooking lends itself well to high fiber eating.

Easy BBQ Chickpea Casserole
So delicious, so nutritious, so quick to prepare.

4 cups cooked or canned chickpeas (two 19-oz cans, drained and rinsed)
2 cups canned stewed tomatoes
3–4 tbsp maple syrup or honey
1 medium onion, chopped
1 green pepper, chopped
1 tsp Dijon mustard
½ tsp cayenne pepper
Freshly ground pepper, to taste

1. Spray a 2-quart ovenproof casserole with nonstick spray. Combine all ingredients and mix well. Cover and bake at 350°F for 1 hour.

Yield: 6 servings. Freezes and/or reheats well. Also excellent served cold.

242 calories per cup, 3.1 g fat (0.3 g saturated), 0 mg cholesterol, 11 g protein, 45 g carbohydrate, 218 mg sodium, 597 mg potassium, 4 mg iron, 10 g fiber, 95 mg calcium

Variations
- Add 1 cup sliced mushrooms. Season with ½ teaspoon each dried basil and thyme.
- Delicious with Vegetarian Stuffed Peppers (page 170).

Easy Enchiladas

1 onion, chopped
1 cup mushrooms, sliced
2 tsp olive oil
2 cloves garlic, crushed
19 oz (540 ml) can kidney beans
1 cup canned or frozen corn, drained
2 cups tomato sauce
¼ tsp red pepper flakes
8 corn or flour tortillas
1 cup grated low-fat cheddar cheese

1. Preheat oven to 350°F. Sauté onion and mushrooms in oil for 5 minutes. Add garlic and cook 2 minutes longer. Rinse and drain beans thoroughly. Place beans in a bowl and mash slightly. Add to skillet along with corn. Add ½ cup of sauce and red pepper flakes; mix well.
2. Spray an oblong Pyrex casserole with nonstick spray. Soften tortillas by heating in the microwave on HIGH about 1 minute. Spread ½ cup sauce in bottom of casserole. Spoon some of bean/corn mixture on each tortilla in a strip across the middle. Roll up tightly and arrange seam side down in casserole. Top with remaining sauce. Cover and bake for 25 minutes. Uncover, sprinkle with cheese and bake uncovered 5 to 10 minutes longer, until cheese is melted.

Yield: 8 enchiladas. These reheat and/or freeze well.

199 calories per serving, 5 g fat (1.1 g saturated), 3 mg cholesterol, 11 g protein, 30 g carbohydrate, 508 mg sodium, 346 mg potassium, 1 mg iron, 5 g fiber, 105 mg calcium

Easy Vegetarian Chili

You won't believe this delicious, high fiber chili contains no meat! Don't be deterred by the long list of ingredients. They're mostly herbs and spices. This chili is quick to prepare and tastes better the next day! Cocoa is the secret ingredient. It deepens the color and rounds out the flavor.

1 tbsp olive or canola oil
2 onions, chopped
2 green and/or red peppers, chopped
3 cloves garlic, crushed
2 cups mushrooms, sliced
2 cups cooked or canned red kidney beans
2 cups cooked or canned chickpeas
½ cup bulgur or couscous, rinsed
28 oz (796 ml) can tomatoes (or 6 fresh tomatoes, chopped)
1 cup bottled salsa (mild or medium)
½ cup water
1 tsp salt (or to taste)
1 tbsp chili powder
1 tsp dried basil
½ tsp each pepper, oregano, and cumin
¼ tsp cayenne
1 tbsp unsweetened cocoa powder
1 tsp sugar
1 cup corn niblets, optional

- *Conventional Method:* Heat oil in a large pot. Sauté onions, peppers, and garlic for 5 minutes on medium heat. Add mushrooms and sauté 4 or 5 minutes more. Add remaining ingredients except corn. Bring to a boil and simmer, covered, for 25 minutes, stirring occasionally. Stir in corn.

- *Microwave Method:* Combine oil, onions, peppers, and garlic in a 3-quart microsafe pot. Microwave covered on HIGH for 5 minutes. Add mushrooms and microwave 2 minutes longer. Add remaining ingredients except corn. Cover and microwave on HIGH for 18 to 20 minutes, stirring once or twice. Add corn. Let stand covered for 10 minutes.

Yield: 10 servings of approximately 1 cup each. Freezes and/or reheats well.

179 calories per serving, 3 g fat (0.4 g saturated), 0 mg cholesterol, 9 g protein, 32 g carbohydrate, 431 mg sodium, 619 mg potassium, 4 mg iron, 9 g fiber, 81 mg calcium

Chef's Secrets
- A 19 oz (540 ml) can of beans or chickpeas contains 2 cups. Rinse well to remove excess sodium.
- **Gluten-Free Chili:** If you are allergic to wheat, do not use bulgur or couscous. Instead, substitute 1 cup of quinoa or millet. Rinse thoroughly and drain well. (Millet requires pretoasting. Cook it on medium heat in a heavy-bottomed skillet about 5 minutes, stirring constantly to prevent burning. It's ready when it gives off a toasty aroma similar to popcorn.) Add to remaining ingredients and cook as directed.
- Serve over rice, noodles, or polenta. Great with Greek Salad (page 189).

Eggplant Roll-Ups
Eggplant replaces pasta in this simple and delicious vegetarian dish. Great for brunch!

1 medium eggplant (do not peel)
10 oz pkg (300 g) frozen spinach, cooked, drained, and squeezed dry
1 cup pressed dry nonfat cottage cheese
3 tbsp grated Parmesan cheese
2 tbsp fresh basil, minced (or 1 tsp dried)
¼ cup skim milk

Salt, pepper, and garlic powder, to taste

2 cups tomato sauce

¾ cup grated low-fat mozzarella cheese

1. Preheat oven to 350°F. Slice eggplant lengthwise into 12 slices, discarding the outer slices. Arrange on a sprayed baking sheet. Bake for 10 minutes, until soft and pliable. Meanwhile, process spinach, cheeses, basil, milk, and seasonings. Mix well. Pour 1 cup of sauce into a sprayed 9- by 13-inch casserole. Spread filling in a thin layer on each slice of eggplant and roll up tightly. Place seam side down in casserole. Top with remaining sauce and sprinkle lightly with cheese. Bake uncovered for 25 to 30 minutes, until golden and bubbling. Perfect with a garden salad.

Yield: 8 rolls. Freezes and/or reheats well. Double the recipe if you have guests.

102 calories per roll, 2.7 g fat (1.6 g saturated), 11 mg cholesterol, 10 g protein, 11 g carbohydrate, 582 mg sodium, 480 mg potassium, 1 mg iron, 3 g fiber, 173 mg calcium

Enchilada Lasagna

No-roll enchiladas are layered like lasagna. Full of fiber and so calci-yummy!

2 tsp olive oil

1 onion, chopped

1-½ cups mushrooms, sliced

1 green pepper, chopped

2 cloves garlic, crushed

3 cups tomato sauce (low-sodium, if possible)

19 oz (540 ml) can kidney beans (rinsed and drained)

½ tsp chili powder (to taste)

7 corn or flour tortillas

¾ cup grated low-fat mozzarella cheese

¾ cup grated low-fat Swiss cheese

1. Preheat oven to 350°F. Heat oil in a nonstick skillet. Sauté veggies and garlic for 5 minutes. Add sauce, beans and chili powder. Simmer uncovered for 5 minutes. Spray a 2-quart casserole with nonstick spray. Layer 2 tortillas, ⅓ of sauce mixture and ⅓ of cheeses, until all ingredients are used, making 3 layers. Cut up the extra tortilla to fill in any empty spaces. Bake uncovered for 25 minutes.

Yield: 6 servings. Reheats and/or freezes well.

273 calories per serving, 5.8 g fat (2.2 g saturated), 13 mg cholesterol, 17 g protein, 41 g carbohydrate, 154 mg sodium, 617 mg potassium, 2 mg iron, 11 g fiber, 288 mg calcium

Italian-Style Baked Tofu

1 lb firm tofu (500 g), sliced ½-inch thick (low-fat tofu can be used)
2 large onions, sliced
1 cup mushrooms, sliced
½ of a red pepper, chopped
½ of a green pepper, chopped
2-½ cups vegetarian spaghetti sauce

1. Place sliced tofu between layers of paper towels on a plate. Top with another plate. Weigh it down with cans and let drain for 20 minutes. Preheat oven to 400°F. Spray a 9- by 13-inch casserole with nonstick spray. Place vegetables in the bottom of the dish. Add half of sauce and mix well. Place tofu on top of vegetable mixture. Top with remaining sauce. Bake uncovered for 40 to 45 minutes, basting once or twice during cooking.

Yield: 6 servings. Serve over pasta. Reheats well. Do not freeze.

213 calories per serving, 10.7 g fat (1.6 g saturated), 0 mg cholesterol, 15 g protein, 20 g carbohydrate, 560 mg sodium, 771 mg potassium, 10 mg iron, 5 g fiber, 192 mg calcium

Kasha Chili

Wholegrain kasha provides a meaty texture to this meatless chili, which only takes 30 minutes to prepare and cook. Steaming hot, fiber-packed kasha chili is sure to take the chill out and warm you up on a cold winter day.

1 can (28 oz/796 ml) diced or stewed tomatoes
3-½ cups vegetable broth
1 can (19 oz/540 ml) black or kidney beans, drained and rinsed
1 large onion, chopped
1 red bell or green pepper, chopped
1 cup sliced mushrooms
2 cloves garlic (about 2 tsp minced)
Salt and freshly ground black pepper
1 tbsp chili powder (or to taste)
1 tbsp unsweetened cocoa powder
1 tsp each paprika, cumin, and oregano
¾ cup whole-grain or medium-grain kasha (buckwheat groats)

1. In a large pot, combine all the ingredients except the kasha and mix well; bring to a boil. Reduce heat to low and simmer, uncovered, for 10 minutes.
2. Stir in the kasha. Cover and simmer for 15 minutes longer or until the kasha is tender, stirring occasionally. If the chili is too thick, thin with a little water. Serve immediately.

Yield: About 8 cups. Keeps for up to 3 to 4 days in the refrigerator; reheats well. Freezes well for up to 3 months.

141 calories per cup, 31.3 g carbohydrate, 7.8 g fiber, 6 g protein, 1.1 g fat (0.2 g saturated), 0 mg cholesterol, 601 mg sodium, 345 mg potassium, 2 mg iron, 63 mg calcium

Variation

- Substitute ½ cup uncooked green or brown lentils for the beans. In Step 1, increase the cooking time to 20 minutes before adding the kasha.

Chef's Secrets

- *Can-Do:* The can from the tomatoes holds 3-½ cups, so measure the vegetable broth right in the empty can.
- *No Yolk-ing!* You don't need an egg to coat the kasha in this recipe. The thin seed coating will shield each kernel while it cooks, keeping it separate and fluffy.

Nutrition Notes

- *Sodium Alert!* If sodium is a concern, choose an organic brand of canned black beans, which usually contains anywhere from 15 to 140 mg of sodium per serving compared to 400 to 480 mg found in regular brands of canned beans. Also, choose low-sodium brands of canned tomatoes and vegetable broth.

Lentil Vegetable Medley

This nutritious dish is jam-packed with fiber and flavor. Delicious over bulgur, quinoa, rotini, or rice, it makes a heart-healthy vegetarian main dish or side dish. Don't be turned off by the long list of ingredients. Just turn on your processor and give it a whirl, girl!

3 cloves garlic (about 1 tbsp minced)
2 medium onions, cut in chunks
2 stalks celery, cut in chunks
3 medium carrots, cut in chunks
1-½ cups mushrooms
2 tbsp olive oil
1 can (28 oz/796 ml) tomatoes (don't drain)
1-½ cups water
2 cups brown or green lentils, drained and rinsed
1 bay leaf
1 tsp Italian seasoning (or a mixture of oregano, basil, and thyme)

Salt and freshly ground black pepper
1 tbsp lemon juice (preferably fresh)
2 tbsp maple syrup or honey
¼ cup minced fresh parsley

1. In a food processor fitted with the steel blade, process the garlic, onions, and celery until chopped, using quick on/off pulses. Transfer the chopped mixture to a bowl. Add the carrots and mushrooms to the food processor and repeat the process, transferring the chopped carrots and mushrooms to the bowl with the rest of the chopped vegetables.
2. In a large pot, heat the oil on medium heat. Add the chopped vegetables and sauté for about 6 to 8 minutes or until tender, stirring occasionally.
3. Add the tomatoes, water, lentils, bay leaf, and Italian seasoning; bring to a boil. Reduce heat to low, partly cover, and simmer for about 1 hour or until the lentils are tender, stirring occasionally. Add a little extra water if needed.
4. Add the salt, pepper, lemon juice, and maple syrup; simmer for 10 minutes longer. Remove the bay leaf, add the parsley, and serve.

Yield: 9 servings of 1 cup each. Tastes even better the next day. Keeps for up to 3 to 4 days in the refrigerator; reheats well. Freezes well for up to 3 months.

232 calories per serving, 39.7 g carbohydrate, 12.1 g fiber, 13 g protein, 3.8 g fat (0.5 g saturated), 0 mg cholesterol, 246 mg sodium, 840 mg potassium, 6 mg iron, 85 mg calcium

Variation

*   *Leftovers?* Transform them into soup. In a saucepan, combine 4 cups of the cooked lentil mixture with 3 cups vegetable broth. Season with salt and pepper and bring to a boil. Reduce heat to low and simmer, partly covered, for 10 minutes. Makes 6 servings.

Pita Pizzas

So quick, so easy, so nutritious! Ideal as an appetizer, or perfect for kids as a quick meal. Pizzas can be topped with tuna, spinach, broccoli, cauliflower, zucchini, Parmesan cheese … have it your way!

2–4 whole-wheat or white pitas (6-½ inch)
½ cup tomato sauce
6 sun-dried tomatoes, rehydrated and cut into strips (or 4 fresh tomatoes, sliced)
½ cup sliced red or green pepper
½ cup sliced mushrooms
¼ cup sliced onion, optional
2 tbsp fresh basil, minced (or ½ tsp dried)
1 cup low-fat grated mozzarella cheese

1. If pitas are thick, split them in half. Place cut-side up on a foil-lined baking sheet. Spread each pita with 2 tablespoons sauce. Add toppings. Bake in a preheated 425°F oven for 10 minutes, or until cheese melts and pizzas are piping hot. As appetizers, cut into 24 wedges with scissors or a pizza wheel.

Yield: 4 pizzas as a main dish or 24 wedges as an appetizer. These freeze and/or reheat well.

189 calories per pizza, 5.9 g fat (3.2 g saturated), 15 mg cholesterol, 12 g protein, 24 g carbohydrate, 576 mg sodium, 372 mg potassium, 2 mg iron, 4 g fiber, 223 mg calcium

Variations

- To rehydrate sun-dried tomatoes: Cover tomatoes with boiling water. Let stand for 10 minutes. (Or cover with cold water and microwave on HIGH for 1 minute. Soak for 5 minutes, until soft.) Drain well. Scissors work well to cut up sun-dried tomatoes.
- As appetizers, each wedge contains 32 calories, 1 g fat (0.5 g saturated), and 3 mg cholesterol.

- **Salsa Pita Pizzas:** Substitute salsa for tomato sauce. If desired, add 2 cloves of thinly sliced garlic. Monterey Jack can be used instead of mozzarella. Bake as directed. Cut into wedges.
- **Pesto Pita Pizzas:** Place pitas on a foil-lined pan. Spread each pita with 1 or 2 tablespoons pesto. Top with strips of roasted red peppers. Allow half of a pepper per pizza. Sprinkle each pita with ¼ cup grated low-fat mozzarella. Bake in a preheated 425°F oven for 10 minutes, until cheese melts. Cut into wedges.
- **Tortilla Pizzas:** In any of the above pizzas, substitute three 9-inch flour tortillas for pitas. Before adding toppings to tortillas, pierce in several places with a fork to prevent them from puffing up. Bake directly on the oven rack in a preheated 400°F oven about 5 minutes, until crisp. Transfer to a foil-lined baking sheet and top with desired toppings. Sprinkle with grated cheese. (Salsa and Monterey Jack cheese are great!) Place under the broiler for a few minutes, until cheese melts. Cut into wedges.

Simple and Good Ratatouille (Mediterranean Vegetable Stew)

2 medium eggplants (2-½ lb/1.2 kg)
2 medium onions
1 green and 1 red pepper
1 medium zucchini
2 cups mushrooms
4 cloves garlic, minced
1–2 tbsp olive oil
Salt and pepper, to taste
½ tsp each dried basil and oregano
¼ cup balsamic or red wine vinegar
2 tbsp brown sugar (to taste)
2 can (5-½ oz/156 ml) tomato paste
½ cup water

165

1. Spray a large, heavy-bottomed pot with nonstick spray. Dice vegetables (do not peel eggplant). Add oil to pot and heat on medium heat. Add vegetables and sauté for 10 to 15 minutes, stirring often. If necessary, add a little water to prevent sticking.
2. Add seasonings, vinegar, brown sugar, tomato paste, and water. Simmer covered for 25 to 30 minutes, stirring occasionally. If mixture gets too thick, add a little water. Adjust seasonings to taste. Serve hot or cold.

Yield: 8 to 10 servings. Mixture keeps up to 10 days in the refrigerator or freezes well.

134 calories per serving, 2.4 g fat (0.4 g saturated), 0 mg cholesterol, 4 g protein, 28 g carbohydrate, 318 mg sodium, 906 mg potassium, 2 mg iron, 6 g fiber, 44 mg calcium

Chef's Secrets

- Delicious over spaghetti squash, rice, bulgur, couscous, polenta, millet, or your favorite grain.
- Ratatouille makes a great vegetarian pasta sauce. Serve it hot over spiral pasta or penne and sprinkle with grated low-fat mozzarella or Parmesan cheese. Heat for 2 minutes in the microwave to melt the cheese.
- Use Ratatouille instead of tomato sauce in lasagna. It also makes a great filling for crêpes. Leftover Ratatouille makes a perfect pizza topping.
- Serve a scoop of chilled Ratatouille on a bed of salad greens as a starter or light main course.
- Serve it cold as an appetizer with Pita or Baked Tortilla Chips (page 342), crackers, or assorted breads.
- **Easy Vegetarian Stew:** In Step 2, add any of the following cut-up vegetables: yellow squash, celery, carrots, potatoes or sweet potatoes, fresh or sun-dried tomatoes, green beans, asparagus. You can also add canned chickpeas, black beans and/or kidney beans, rinsed and drained. If desired, dice ½ lb (250 g) of tofu and add to stew mixture during the last 10 minutes of cooking. (Tofu that was frozen, then thawed, will have a meaty texture.) Serve over rice, bulgur, pasta, couscous, or polenta.

Terrific Tofu Stir-Fry

This yummy, versatile dish is equally delicious with chicken or tofu! Calci-yummy!

Tofu and Marinade:

1 lb firm tofu (500 g), sliced into ½-inch slices

¼ cup vegetable or pareve chicken broth

3 tbsp soy sauce

2 tbsp rice or white wine vinegar

1 tsp sugar

1 tbsp grated ginger

2 cloves garlic, crushed

Vegetables:

3 cups broccoli florets

2 tbsp sesame seeds

1 tbsp peanut or canola oil

2 red peppers, cut into strips

1 cup green onions, sliced

3 cloves garlic, crushed

1 tbsp grated ginger

2 cups mushrooms, sliced

½ lb fresh spinach, in bite-sized pieces

2 cups bean sprouts

2 tsp Oriental sesame oil

¼ tsp red pepper flakes (crushed chilis)

½ tbsp cornstarch dissolved in ¼ cup orange juice or broth

1. Place tofu between paper towels on a plate. Top with another plate, weigh down with cans and let stand for 20 minutes. Cut into ½-inch strips. Combine all marinade ingredients. Add tofu and marinate for 30 minutes, or refrigerate covered overnight, basting occasionally.

2. Cook broccoli until bright green but still crunchy. (Microwave covered on HIGH for 2 minutes or boil for 2 or 3 minutes.) Rinse immediately in cold water; drain and set aside. In a wok, toast sesame seeds until golden, shaking pan to prevent burning. Remove from pan; set aside. Add oil to wok. Stir-fry peppers and green onions on high for 1 minute. Add garlic, ginger, and mushrooms; stir-fry for 2 minutes.

3. Stir in tofu, marinade, broccoli, spinach, and sprouts. Reduce heat to medium, cover and cook for 2 minutes, until heated through. Stir in sesame oil, red pepper flakes, and cornstarch mixture. Bring to a boil and stir until thickened. Sprinkle with sesame seeds.

Yield: 8 servings. Serve over steamed rice or noodles. Do not freeze.

169 calories per serving, 9.3 g fat (1.3 g saturated), 0 mg cholesterol, 13 g protein, 12 g carbohydrate, 415 mg sodium, 510 mg potassium, 8 mg iron, 4 g fiber, 186 mg calcium

Variations

- Use leftover broccoli stems in your favorite vegetable soup. Chinese greens, pea pods, sliced green peppers, and/or partially cooked carrots can be added or substituted in the above recipe.
- **Chicken Stir-Fry:** Substitute 2 lbs boneless, skinless chicken breasts, cut in ½-inch strips. In Step 2, stir-fry chicken 2 to 3 minutes. Add peppers, ginger, and green onions; complete recipe as directed. One serving contains 208 calories, 7 g fat (1.3 saturated) and 63 mg cholesterol.

Vegetarian Cabbage Rolls

Whether you call these Halishkes or Prakkes, they taste great!

Rainbow Rice Pilaf (page 218)
1 medium cabbage (about 3 lb/1.2 kg)
Boiling water
19 oz can (540 ml) tomatoes
5-½ oz can (156 ml) tomato paste

¼ cup brown sugar, packed

2 tbsp lemon juice

1 large onion, chopped

1. Prepare Rainbow Rice Pilaf as directed; let cool. Meanwhile, remove 12 of the large outer leaves from cabbage. Trim away tough ribs. Place cabbage leaves into a large pot of boiling water. Remove pot from heat, cover and let stand for 10 minutes. Drain cabbage thoroughly and set aside.

2. In the same pot, combine tomatoes, tomato paste, brown sugar, and lemon juice. Break up tomatoes with a spoon. Remove ½ cup of sauce from pot and add it to rice mixture. Mix well.

3. Bring sauce mixture to a boil. Slice any leftover cabbage and add it to the sauce along with the chopped onion. Meanwhile, place a large spoonful of rice mixture on each cabbage leaf. Roll up, folding in ends. Carefully place cabbage rolls seam-side down in simmering sauce. Cook on low heat, partially covered, about 1 hour, until juice has thickened. Adjust seasonings to taste.

Yield: 12 cabbage rolls. These reheat well. Freezing is not recommended.

159 calories per cabbage roll, 1.7 g fat (0.2 g saturated), 0 mg cholesterol, 5 g protein, 34 g carbohydrate, 372 mg sodium, 479 mg potassium, 2 mg iron, 5 g fiber, 70 mg calcium

Variations

- Crushed or diced canned tomatoes can be used. If you only have a very large can of tomatoes on hand, either freeze the leftovers or add them to your next vegetable soup or pasta sauce!
- *Veggie Variations:* If you have frozen tofu on hand, defrost and crumble it. You'll need about 1 cup. Combine crumbled tofu with rice mixture. Add salt, pepper, and basil to taste. Stuff cabbage as directed. Another variation is to add 1 cup cooked or canned lentils or chickpeas.
- For other ideas for fillings, see notes following Vegetarian Stuffed Peppers (page 170).

Vegetarian Stuffed Peppers

Easy, delicious and colorful.

Rainbow Rice Pilaf (page 218)
6 peppers (green, red, yellow, and/or orange)
4 cups water
1-½ cups tomato sauce (bottled or homemade)

1. Prepare Rainbow Rice Pilaf as directed, using vegetable broth. Cut
    peppers in half lengthwise through stem end. Carefully remove seeds and
    core. In a large saucepan, bring water to a boil. Add peppers and simmer
    for 3 or 4 minutes, until slightly softened. Drain well. Preheat oven to
    350°F. Fill peppers with rice mixture. Spread 1 cup sauce on the bottom
    of a sprayed Pyrex oblong casserole. Arrange peppers in a single layer
    over sauce. Drizzle lightly with remaining sauce. Bake uncovered for 25
    minutes (or microwave uncovered on HIGH for 12 to 15 minutes), until
    peppers are tender and heated through.

Yield: 6 servings as a main dish or 12 servings as a side dish. Reheats well. Do
not freeze.

*232 calories per main dish serving, 2.5 g fat (0.4 g saturated), 0 mg cholesterol,
7 g protein, 48 g carbohydrate, 727 mg sodium, 586 mg potassium, 3 mg iron, 5 g
fiber, 52 mg calcium*

Variations

• Add ½ cup diced tofu to cooked rice for additional protein. For
  additional soluble fiber, add ½ cup canned red kidney beans or chickpeas, rinsed and drained. For additional calcium and protein, top each
  pepper with 2 tablespoons grated low-fat Swiss, Parmesan, or mozzarella
  cheese during the last 10 minutes of baking (or last 5 minutes of
  microwaving).

- *Stuffed Vegetables:* Any of the above fillings can be used to stuff Vegetarian Cabbage Rolls (page 168). Other veggies that are lovely when stuffed are hollowed-out tomatoes, zucchini, or yellow squash halves. Use your imagination!

Winter Vegetable Stew

My cousin Carol Teichman, of Toronto, shared this recipe for her hearty vegetable stew, and I've modified it slightly to speed up the preparation. Don't stew over the long list of ingredients—this comes together very quickly. Chop the vegetables in batches in your food processor, and add them to the pot as they are ready. This scrumptious stew is sure to warm you up on a cold winter day.

2 tbsp olive or canola oil
2 large onions, chopped
2 stalks celery, chopped
2 cloves garlic (about 2 tsp minced)
2 medium carrots, chopped (or 12 baby carrots)
2 parsnips, peeled and chopped
2 medium potatoes, cut into 1-inch cubes, or 6 small new potatoes
2 cups green beans, trimmed and sliced into 1-inch pieces
1 red pepper, seeded and coarsely chopped
2 cups sliced mushrooms
1 to 2 tbsp chopped fresh dillweed or 1 tsp dried
1 tsp dried oregano
2-½ cups vegetable broth
1 tbsp Dijon mustard
1 tbsp maple syrup
Salt and freshly ground black pepper

1. Heat the oil in a large, heavy-bottomed pot over medium heat. Add the onions and celery, and sauté for 6 to 8 minutes or until golden.

2. Stir in the garlic, carrots, parsnips, potatoes, and green beans; mix well. Cook for 2 to 3 minutes. Add the red pepper and mushrooms and cook for 2 minutes before adding the dillweed, oregano, and broth; bring to a boil.

3. Reduce heat to low and stir in the mustard and maple syrup. Simmer for 10 to 12 minutes or until the potatoes are just tender. Season with salt and pepper to taste.

Yield: 6 servings. Keeps for up to 2 to 3 days in the refrigerator; reheats well. Don't freeze.

204 calories per serving, 37.4 g carbohydrate, 6.8 g fiber, 4 g protein, 5.5 g fat (0.7 g saturated), 0 mg cholesterol, 501 mg sodium, 712 mg potassium, 2 mg iron, 84 mg calcium

Nutrition Notes

- For additional protein, add 1 to 2 cups of black, navy, or red kidney beans (canned are fine, but drain and rinse well) in Step 2, along with the vegetables. Or add 1 cup diced, extra-firm tofu.
- For another protein boost, serve with an assortment of low-fat cheeses such as cheddar, Swiss, or havarti, and pumpernickel bread.

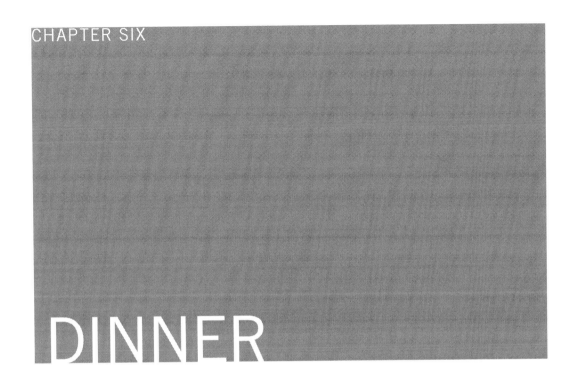

CHAPTER SIX

DINNER

■ SOUPS

Bean and vegetable soups are full of fiber, and they're filling. Try them as a main course with high fiber bread and a salad.

Autumn Vegetable Soup
(See recipe, page 70)

Bean, Barley and Sweet Potato Soup
(See recipe, page 72)

Black Bean, Barley and Vegetable Soup
Black beans are easier to digest than other beans, are very high in antioxidants, and are a good source of protein. This high fiber soup is enhanced with fresh herbs—it's "soup-herb"! (Don't let the long list of ingredients deter you. To save prep time, use a food processor to chop the vegetables.)

    1 to 2 tbsp olive oil
    3 cloves garlic (about 1 tbsp minced)
    2 medium onions, chopped
    2 stalks celery, chopped
    10 cups water, vegetable, or chicken broth
    3 medium carrots, chopped (or 12 baby carrots)
    1-½ cups mushrooms, chopped
    1 medium sweet potato or 2 medium potatoes, peeled and chopped
    ½ cup pearl barley, rinsed and drained
    1 cup dried red lentils, rinsed and drained
    1 can (19 oz/540 ml) black beans, drained and rinsed
    2 tsp salt (or to taste)
    1 tsp freshly ground black pepper (or to taste)
    ¼ cup minced fresh dillweed and/or finely chopped fresh basil
    ¼ cup minced fresh parsley

1. Heat the oil in a large soup pot on medium heat. Add the garlic, onions, and celery, and sauté for 5 to 7 minutes or until golden. If the vegetables start to stick, add 2 to 3 tbsp water.
2. Add the water or broth, carrots, mushrooms, sweet potato, barley, lentils, black beans, salt, and pepper; bring to a boil. Reduce heat and simmer, partially covered, for 1 hour or until the vegetables are tender, stirring occasionally. If the soup becomes too thick, thin with a little water.
3. Add the dillweed and parsley, and adjust the seasonings to taste before serving.

Yield: 8 to 10 servings (about 15 cups). Leftovers keep 4 or 5 days in the refrigerator; reheats well. Freezes well for up to 4 months.

116 calories per cup, 22 g carbohydrate, 5.5 g fiber, 6 g protein, 1.3 g fat (0.2 g saturated), 0 mg cholesterol, 317 mg sodium, 340 mg potassium, 2 mg iron, 36 mg calcium

Nutrition Notes
- Black beans, barley, and lentils all have a low glycemic index, making this soup an excellent choice for diabetics or those who are insulin-resistant.
- Canned black beans are more convenient than dried because you don't need to soak and cook them, but they are higher in sodium. To lower the sodium, choose organic brands of canned black beans, which contain a fraction of the sodium of regular canned beans.

Black Bean Soup
(See recipe, page 73)

Broccoli and Red Pepper Soup
(See recipe, page 74)

Curried Carrot and Cashew Soup

This scrumptious vegetarian soup will fill you up without filling you out! Jackie Toledano of Netanya, Israel, often makes this soup for her family for Friday night dinners. Her children go nuts over it!

1 tbsp olive oil
1 large onion, chopped
1 large apple, peeled, cored, and chopped
1 medium sweet potato or 1 medium potato, peeled and chopped
2 lb (1 kg) baby carrots or frozen baby carrots
8 cups vegetable broth
⅓ cup roasted cashews
1 to 2 tsp salt (or to taste)
½ tsp freshly ground black pepper
1 to 2 tsp curry powder
¼ tsp chili powder
Chopped cashews, for garnish (optional)

1. Heat the oil in a large soup pot on medium high heat. Add the onion, apple, sweet potato, and carrots, and sauté for 5 to 7 minutes or until the vegetables are tender.
2. Add the broth, cashews, salt, and pepper, and bring to a boil. Reduce heat to low and simmer, partially covered, for 30 minutes or until the vegetables are tender. Remove from heat and cool slightly.
3. Using an immersion blender, purée the soup while still in the pot, or purée in batches in a blender or food processor. If the soup is too thick, add a little extra broth or water. (Milk or soymilk are also good choices.) Stir in the curry powder and chili powder and serve hot. Sprinkle with chopped cashews, if desired.

Yield: 6 to 8 servings (about 12 cups). Keeps 3 to 4 days in the refrigerator; reheats well. Freezes well for up to 4 months.

112 calories per cup, 18.7 g carbohydrate, 3.6 g fiber, 3 g protein, 3.3 g fat (0.5 g saturated), 0 mg cholesterol, 546 mg sodium, 91 mg potassium, 1 mg iron, 41 mg calcium

Variations

- **Dill Carrot Cashew Soup:** Instead of curry and chili powder, substitute with 2 tbsp minced fresh dillweed, adding it at the end of the cooking process.
- *Nut-Free Variation:* Replace cashews with 1 medium turnip or squash, peeled and coarsely chopped.

Chef's Secrets

- *A-Peeling News!* Instead of using raw baby carrots or frozen carrots, use 2 lb (1 kg) regular carrots, peeled and coarsely chopped. (Jackie and I both prefer the lazy method—no peeling or cutting required.)
- *Cash in on Cashews:* Store cashews in a tightly sealed container in the refrigerator for up to 6 months or freeze them for up to a year. No cashews? Use blanched almonds.

Easy Corn Chowder
(See recipe, page 76)

Luscious Lentil Soup
(See recipe, page 77)

Mango Gazpacho

Ladle up some sunshine with this colorful chilled soup, packed with vitamin A, beta carotene, and potassium: it's "mang"-nificent! Serve in wine glasses or champagne flutes for an elegant presentation.

3 to 4 cloves garlic (about 1 tbsp minced)
1 medium red onion, cut in chunks (about 1 cup)
2 mangoes, peeled, pitted, and cut in chunks (about 2 cups)

2 tbsp fresh basil
¼ cup lightly packed fresh cilantro leaves
1 unpeeled English cucumber, cut in chunks
1 red pepper, seeded and cut in chunks
2 Roma tomatoes, cut in chunks
1 tbsp extra virgin olive oil
2 tbsp lemon juice (preferably fresh)
2 tbsp lime juice (preferably fresh)
1 tsp salt (or to taste)
¼ tsp freshly ground black pepper
¾ to 1 tsp chili powder
2 cups orange juice or 1 cup mango and 1 cup orange juice

1. Drop the garlic through the feed tube of the food processor while the motor is running; process until minced. Add the onion, mangoes, basil, and cilantro; process with quick on/off pulses, until finely chopped. Transfer to a large mixing bowl.
2. In the food processor, process the cucumber, red pepper, and tomatoes with quick on/off pulses, until finely chopped.
3. Add to the mango mixture along with the oil, lemon and lime juices, salt, pepper, and chili powder. Stir in the orange juice, cover and refrigerate until serving time.

Yield: 5 to 6 servings (about 7 cups). Keeps 2 days in the refrigerator. Don't freeze.

115 calories per cup, 23.8 g carbohydrate, 2.3 g fiber, 2 g protein, 2.6 g fat (0.4 g saturated), 0 mg cholesterol, 340 mg sodium, 416 mg potassium, 1 mg iron, 33 mg calcium

Mighty Minestrone
(See recipe, page 79)

Red Lentil, Vegetable and Barley Soup

1 tbsp olive or canola oil
3 large onions, chopped
4 cloves garlic, minced
¼ cup fresh parsley, minced
4 stalks celery, chopped
6 carrots, coarsely chopped
1 large sweet potato, peeled and chopped
2 zucchini, ends trimmed, chopped
10 cups water, chicken or vegetable broth
1-½ cups red lentils, rinsed and drained
½ cup pearl barley, rinsed and drained
1 tbsp salt (or to taste)
½ tsp pepper
1 tsp dried basil (or 1 tbsp fresh)
2 tbsp fresh dill, minced

1. Heat oil in a large soup pot. Add garlic and onions. Sauté on medium heat until golden, about 5 to 7 minutes. Add a little water if vegetables begin to stick. Add remaining ingredients. Bring to a boil, reduce heat and simmer partly covered for 1 hour, or until barley is tender. Stir occasionally. Thin with a little water if soup is too thick. Adjust seasonings to taste.

Yield: 12 servings.

169 calories per serving, 1.7 g fat (0.3 g saturated), 0 mg cholesterol, 8 g protein, 32 g carbohydrate, 629 mg sodium, 530 mg potassium, 3 mg iron, 10 g fiber, 55 mg calcium

Red Lentil, Zucchini and Couscous Soup
(See recipe, page 82)

Secret Ingredient Cabbage Borscht

Bagged coleslaw mix is the secret ingredient to help speed up preparation for this scrumptious soup. Most of the ingredients are probably in your kitchen. Big soup, little effort!

2 tbsp olive or canola oil
3 medium onions, chopped
1 pkg (16 oz/500 g) coleslaw mix
3 cloves garlic (about 1 tbsp minced)
8 cups water, vegetable or chicken broth
1 cup tomato juice
1 can (28 oz/796 ml) diced or whole tomatoes, undrained
1 can (5½ oz/156 ml) tomato paste
1 cup dried green, brown, or red lentils, rinsed and drained
¼ cup brown sugar or granular Splenda (or to taste)
½ tsp freshly ground black pepper
1 bay leaf
2 tsp salt (or to taste)
2 tbsp lemon juice (preferably fresh)
2 tbsp minced fresh dillweed

1. In a large soup pot, heat the oil on medium heat. Add the onions and sauté for 5 minutes or until tender. Add the coleslaw mix and garlic, and cook 5 to 7 minutes longer or until tender, stirring occasionally.
2. Stir in the water, tomato juice, tomatoes, tomato paste, lentils, brown sugar, pepper, and bay leaf, and bring to a boil. Reduce the heat and simmer, partially covered, for 1-½ hours or until the lentils are tender. If the soup gets too thick, add a little water or broth.
3. Stir in the salt, lemon juice, and dillweed; simmer 5 minutes longer to blend the flavors. Remove and discard the bay leaf before serving.

Yield: 8 to 10 servings (about 16 cups). Keeps 3 to 4 days in the refrigerator; reheats well. Freezes well for up to 4 months.

103 calories per cup, 18.1 g carbohydrate, 3.6 g fiber, 4 g protein, 2.0 g fat (0.3 g saturated), 0 mg cholesterol, 539 mg sodium, 264 mg potassium, 1 mg iron, 33 mg calcium

Chef's Secrets

- *Grate Idea!* Instead of coleslaw mix, substitute 6 cups grated cabbage and 1 grated carrot. If you want to include more vegetables, add 2 stalks chopped celery and 1 chopped zucchini.
- *Color Your World!* Green or brown dried lentils will retain their shape, whereas red dried lentils will disintegrate during cooking and disappear into the soup.
- *Juicy News:* Always add salt and lemon juice at the end of the cooking time to soups containing beans or lentils. If you add them at the start of the cooking process, the lentils won't soften completely.
- *Sodi-Yum!* If you are concerned about sodium, use sodium-free tomato juice, canned tomatoes, and tomato paste.

Split Pea and Portobello Mushroom Soup

This decadent, velvety soup is full of fiber and flavor. My walking partner, Frieda Wishinsky, uses shallots rather than garlic in her cooking because they add another dimension of flavor. Frieda, a children's book author, refers to herself as "The Lady of Shallots." I'm sure Lord Tennyson would have poetic praise for her heavenly soup.

1 cup dried green split peas, rinsed and drained
5 cups water
1 cup vegetable or chicken broth
1 tbsp canola or olive oil
1 large sweet onion, chopped
2 medium shallots (about ½ cup chopped)
2 cups sliced portobello mushrooms (about 5 mushrooms)
1 medium carrot, chopped

¼ tsp paprika (sweet or smoked)
1 tsp salt
Freshly ground black pepper

1. Combine the split peas, water, and broth in a large pot. Bring to a boil. Reduce the heat to low, cover partially, and simmer for 35 minutes.
2. While the peas are cooking, heat the oil in a large skillet on medium-high heat. Add the onion, shallots, and mushrooms, and sauté until golden brown, about 5 minutes. Reduce the heat and cook slowly until the onion has caramelized, about 5 to 10 minutes.
3. Add the onion mixture to the peas. Add the carrot and simmer 15 minutes longer or until tender. Stir in the paprika and remove from heat to let cool slightly.
4. Using an immersion blender, purée the soup while still in the pot or purée in batches in a blender or food processor. If too thick, add a little water or broth. Season with salt and pepper to taste, and serve.

Yield: 4 to 5 servings (about 7 cups). Keeps 3 to 4 days in the refrigerator; reheats well. Freezes well for up to 4 months. If too thick, add a little water when reheating.

123 calories per cup, 19.6 g carbohydrate, 6.7 g fiber, 7 g protein, 2.4 g fat (0.2 g saturated), 0 mg cholesterol, 411 mg sodium, 376 mg potassium, 1 mg iron, 26 mg calcium

Variations

- Use a combination of split peas and lentils. You can use either green or yellow split peas.
- Cook ¼ cup pearl barley, rinsed and drained, along with peas and/or lentils. Or substitute barley for half the peas. This makes a thicker soup, so thin as needed with additional broth.
- No shallots? Use 2 or 3 cloves garlic. Shallots look like small elongated onions, with a garlic flavor. When peeled, they divide into cloves like garlic.
- Instead of portobellos, try shiitake, oyster, or button mushrooms, or a combination of these.

Nutrition Notes

- Split peas are a nutritional powerhouse. Packed with protein, fiber, and vitamin C, they also contain iron, zinc, and B vitamins. Both green and yellow split peas have a low glycemic index (32). Soaking before cooking isn't necessary. A thorough rinsing in a colander is sufficient. When cooked, split peas break down to make a thick, satisfying soup.

Squish Squash Soup

Thanks to my friend Jeff Goodman for this yummy, nutritious soup, which he often serves to guests. Everyone loves it, especially me!

1 medium butternut squash (about 3 lb/1.5 kg) (or 7 to 8 cups frozen squash cubes)

4 cups vegetable broth

6 large mushrooms (about 1 cup sliced)

2 tbsp soy sauce (low-sodium or regular)

½ cup skim milk

½ cup light cream (10% or 5%)

Salt and freshly ground black pepper

1. If using fresh squash, cut in half with a sharp knife and scoop out the seeds (see Chef's Secrets, page 184). Cut into cubes. Combine squash, broth, mushrooms, and soy sauce in a large saucepan; bring to a boil.
2. Reduce heat and simmer, partially covered or until the squash is tender, about 20 minutes. Remove from heat and cool slightly.
3. Using an immersion blender, purée the soup while still in the pot, or purée in batches in a blender or food processor. Stir in milk and cream. Season with salt and pepper to taste, and serve.

Yield: 6 servings (about 8 cups). Keeps 3 days in the refrigerator; reheats well. Freezes well for up to 3 months. Don't boil when reheating or the soup may curdle.

150 calories per cup, 32.3 g carbohydrate, 5.4 g fiber, 4 g protein, 2.1 g fat (1.0 g saturated), 5 mg cholesterol, 484 mg sodium, 913 mg potassium, 2 mg iron, 161 mg calcium

Dairy-Free Variation

- Instead of milk or cream, substitute soymilk.

Toasted Squash Seeds

- Rinse the seeds to remove fibers; pat dry with paper towels. Spread in a single layer on a parchment-lined baking sheet, drizzle with a little olive oil, and sprinkle lightly with salt. Roast, uncovered, at 250°F for about 45 to 60 minutes or until they are toasted and golden, stirring every 20 minutes. The toasted seeds will keep for several months in a sealed container in a cool, dark place. They're ideal as a snack or garnish.

Chef's Secret

- *Short Cuts!* Score the outer skin of a squash with a sharp knife in several places. Microwave, uncovered, for 4 to 5 minutes on high; turn the squash over halfway through cooking. Let stand for 5 minutes or until cool enough to handle. The squash will be slightly softened and easier (and safer!) to cut in half. Scoop out the stringy fiber and seeds.

White Bean Soup

Canned beans save on cooking time and the food processor makes quick work of preparing the ingredients. Lemon juice really adds a flavor boost. This recipe can be halved easily, but it's so delicious, why bother? Bean cuisine will keep you lean and healthy, and has a low glycemic index.

3 or 4 cloves garlic (about 1 tbsp minced)
2 medium onions, cut in chunks
2 medium stalks celery, cut in chunks
2 medium carrots, cut in chunks

1 tbsp olive or canola oil
2 cans (19 oz/540 ml each) white kidney beans, drained and rinsed
4 cups vegetable or chicken broth
1 can (28 oz/796 ml) tomatoes (don't drain)
½ tsp dried thyme
1 tsp ground cumin or dried basil
Salt and freshly ground black pepper
2 tbsp lemon juice (preferably fresh)

1. Drop the garlic through the feed tube of a food processor while the motor is running; process until minced, about 10 seconds. Add the onions, celery, and carrots; process with several quick on/off pulses, or until the vegetables are coarsely chopped.
2. Heat the oil in a large soup pot on medium heat. Sauté the vegetables about 5 to 7 minutes or until tender. If they begin to stick, stir in a little water.
3. Working in batches, process the beans together with some of the broth in the food processor until puréed, about 30 seconds. Add to the soup pot. Purée the tomatoes in batches; add them to the pot, along with the seasonings. Bring to a boil; reduce heat to low and simmer, partially covered, for 20 minutes. Stir occasionally.
4. Add the lemon juice, adjust seasonings to taste, and serve.

Yield: 7 to 8 servings (about 12 cups). Keeps 3 to 4 days in the refrigerator; reheats well. Freezes well for up to 4 months.

109 calories per cup, 20.1 g carbohydrate, 4 g fiber, 5 g protein, 1.7 g fat (0.2 g saturated), 0 mg cholesterol, 334 mg sodium, 444 mg potassium, 3 mg iron, 79 mg calcium

Variation
- Instead of beans, substitute canned lentils.

■ SALADS AND DRESSINGS

Avoid salads that are made mostly of lettuce, as lettuce contains little fiber. Vegetable salads, or lettuce salads that are loaded with vegetables and beans, are a better choice. Pair these salads with a cup of bean soup, and you have a fiber-filled meal.

Apricot Hoisin Spinach Salad
(See recipe, page 83)

Balsamic Vinaigrette
(See recipe, page 84)

Best Green Bean Salad
(See recipe, page 85)

Carrot Almond Salad
(See recipe, page 86)

Couscous, Cranberry and Mango Salad
(See recipe, page 87)

Creamy 1,000 Island Cole Slaw
(See recipe, page 88)

Doug's "Flower Power" Cæsar Salad
(See recipe, page 89)

Easy Lentil Salad

2 can (19 oz /540 ml) lentils, rinsed and drained (or 4 cups cooked brown lentils)
2 cloves garlic, minced
1 red or yellow pepper, chopped
1 orange pepper, chopped
2 carrots, grated
6 green onions, chopped
¼ cup minced parsley
2 tbsp extra virgin olive oil
3 tbsp lemon juice
Salt and pepper, to taste
½ tsp each chili powder, dry mustard, and cumin

1. Combine all ingredients in a large bowl and mix well. Season to taste. Cover and refrigerate.

Yield: 8 servings. This salad will keep in the refrigerator for up to 3 days if tightly covered.

173 calories per serving, 4.1 g fat (0.6 g saturated), 0 mg cholesterol, 10 g protein, 26 g carbohydrate, 247 mg sodium, 551 mg potassium, 4 mg iron, 9 g fiber, 41 mg calcium

Variations

- **Kidney Bean and Chickpea Salad:** Instead of lentils, substitute 1 can of red kidney beans and 1 can of chickpeas, rinsed and drained.
- **Quick Couscous Salad:** Omit lentils; substitute 2 cups of couscous. Add 4 cups of water or chicken broth. Let stand for 10 minutes to absorb liquid. Add remaining ingredients; mix well.
- Instead of chili powder, dry mustard, and cumin, add 3 to 4 tablespoons minced basil. Add ½ cup chopped roasted red peppers and ½ cup chopped sun-dried tomatoes to either version of the above salad.

Fattouche Salad
(See recipe, page 90)

Fennel, Orange and Spinach Salad

Fennel, also known as finocchio, has a mild licorice flavor. The fronds (leaves) resemble fresh dill.

> 1 medium bulb fennel (about ½ lb)
> ½ of a 10 oz pkg of fresh spinach
> 4 large seedless oranges
> 1 red pepper, halved, seeded, and thinly sliced
> ½ cup chopped red onion (or 4 green onions)
> 2 tbsp lemon juice or rice vinegar
> 1 clove garlic, crushed
> 1 tsp honey-style mustard
> 2 tbsp extra virgin olive oil
> Salt and pepper, to taste

1. Wash fennel; remove any stringy or brown outer stalks. Chop some of the fronds and reserve. Trim away root end. Slice fennel bulbs and stems into ¼-inch slices and place in a serving bowl. Trim away tough stems from spinach. Wash spinach, dry well and tear into bite-size pieces. Peel oranges with a sharp knife, removing the white pith. Cut in half and slice thinly. Combine oranges in a bowl with fennel, spinach, red pepper, and onion. Refrigerate until serving time. In a small bowl, combine lemon juice, garlic, and mustard. Whisk in oil; refrigerate.
2. At serving time, pour dressing over fennel mixture and toss to coat with dressing. Season with salt and pepper. Garnish with fennel fronds.

Yield: 8 servings. So refreshing!

95 calories per serving, 3.7 g fat (0.5 g saturated), 0 mg cholesterol, 2 g protein, 16 g carbohydrate, 34 mg sodium, 398 mg potassium, <1 mg iron, 4 g fiber, 68 mg calcium

Chef's Secrets

• To test fennel for freshness, press the flesh lightly with your thumb. Avoid any bulbs that are soft.

• **Turkey, Fennel and Orange Salad:** Turn this salad into a main course by topping it with 2 cups of julienned smoked turkey (or chicken).

Greek Chickpea Salad

(See recipe, page 91)

Greek Salad

I've reduced the fat content considerably for this marvelous Mediterranean salad, but not the flavor! It's perfect for a buffet. Double or triple the recipe for a large crowd since it disappears so quickly.

4 firm, ripe tomatoes
3 green peppers (or 1 green, 1 red, 1 yellow)
1 English cucumber, peeled
½ of a red or Spanish onion (about 1 cup)
¼ cup pitted black olives
½ cup feta cheese, finely diced or grated
2 tbsp olive oil (preferably extra virgin)
Juice of a lemon (3 tbsp)
Salt and pepper, to taste
½ tsp each dried basil and oregano

1. Cut tomatoes, peppers, cucumber, and onion into 1-inch chunks. Slice olives or cut them in half. Combine all ingredients in a large bowl and toss to mix. (Can be prepared several hours in advance and refrigerated.)

Yield: 6 servings of about 1 cup each. Leftovers keep for 1–2 days in the refrigerator.

136 calories per serving, 8.5 g fat (2.7 g saturated), 11 mg cholesterol, 4 g protein, 13 g carbohydrate, 202 mg sodium, 473 mg potassium, 1 mg iron, 3 g fiber, 93 mg calcium

Variation

- *Lactose-Free:* Substitute extra-firm tofu (preferably lite) for feta cheese. Slice tofu; place slices between 2 layers of paper towels. Cover with a baking sheet and top with several cans to press out excess liquid. Let stand 20 minutes. Dice tofu and add to salad. Add 2 to 3 tbsp of Parmesan-flavored soy or rice cheese. Toss gently to mix.

Greek-Style Black Bean Salad

So colorful, so good! Silken tofu can be substituted for the feta cheese for a non-dairy version.

2 cans (19 oz/540 ml) black beans, rinsed and drained (or 4 cups cooked)
¾ cup chopped red onion
1 yellow pepper, chopped
1 red pepper, chopped
2–3 tbsp extra virgin olive oil
3 tbsp fresh lemon juice
¼ cup fresh mint leaves, minced
¼ cup fresh parsley leaves, minced
Salt and freshly ground pepper, to taste
2 firm tomatoes, chopped
½ cup feta cheese, crumbled

1. Combine all ingredients except tomatoes and cheese; mix well. Marinate for at least 20 to 30 minutes. Adjust seasonings to taste and garnish with tomatoes and cheese just before serving.

Yield: 8 servings.

199 calories per serving, 6.9 g fat (1.9 g saturated), 8 mg cholesterol, 11 g protein, 26 g carbohydrate, 585 mg sodium, 185 mg potassium, 4 mg iron, 9 g fiber, 107 mg calcium

Honey Mustard Carrot Salad

2 lb carrots, peeled and grated
4 green onions, chopped
2 tbsp chopped parsley and/or dill
3 tbsp honey
1 tbsp Dijon mustard (to taste)
1 tbsp extra virgin olive oil
⅓ cup raisins, rinsed and drained
1 tbsp orange juice
1 tbsp lemon juice
Salt and pepper, to taste

1. Combine all ingredients in a bowl and toss to mix. Adjust seasonings to taste. Serve chilled.

Yield: 6 servings.

115 calories per serving, 2.2 g fat (0.3 g saturated), 0 mg cholesterol, 2 g protein, 25 g carbohydrate, 90 mg sodium, 454 mg potassium, <1 mg iron, 4 g fiber, 43 mg calcium

Indonesian Brown Rice Salad
(See recipe, page 92)

Jodi's Famous Bean Salad
(See recipe, page 94)

Lauren's Black Bean Salad
(See recipe, page 95)

Lighter Cæsar Salad Dressing
(See recipe, page 96)

Luscious Layered Salad

This colorful, nutrition-packed salad tastes just as good as it looks. Thanks to my friend Bella Borts, of Toronto, for sharing this super recipe, which I modified slightly. It's a real crowd-pleaser!

Dressing:
¼ cup rice or cider vinegar
¼ cup extra virgin olive oil
2 cloves garlic (about 2 tsp minced)
1 tsp sea or Kosher salt
¼ tsp freshly ground black pepper
1 tsp dried basil or 2 tbsp chopped fresh
1 tsp dried oregano or 1 tbsp chopped fresh

Salad:
1 can (19 oz/540 ml) black beans, drained and rinsed
1 can (12 oz/341 ml) corn kernels, drained
1 red pepper, halved, seeded, and sliced
½ red onion, halved and sliced
2 cups broccoli or cauliflower florets
1 can (19 oz/540 ml) red kidney beans or chickpeas, drained and rinsed
2 cups chopped tomatoes or 1 container (550 g/1 pint) grape tomatoes
4 cups packed baby spinach leaves or mixed salad greens
½ cup dried cranberries or raisins
½ cup toasted sliced almonds

1. Combine the ingredients for salad dressing in a jar; cover tightly and shake well. Refrigerate until serving time.
2. In a large glass salad bowl, arrange the ingredients in layers, starting with the black beans and ending with the spinach. Top with the cranberries and almonds. Cover and refrigerate for up to 24 hours before serving.
3. At serving time, drizzle the salad dressing over the salad and toss gently to combine. Serve chilled.

Yield: 16 servings (about 1 cup per serving).

137 calories per serving, 19.8 g carbohydrate, 5.7 g fiber, 5 g protein, 5.3 g fat (0.6 g saturated), 0 mg cholesterol, 399 mg sodium, 307 mg potassium, 3 mg iron, 40 mg calcium

Variations

- Add ½ cup thinly sliced or grated carrots, zucchini, and/or sliced mushrooms. Instead of dried cranberries or raisins, substitute dried blueberries. Instead of almonds, top with chopped pistachios or roasted soy nuts.

Chef's Secrets

- *I Be Leaf!* If using flat-leaf spinach, wash it well, dry thoroughly, and tear into bite-sized pieces.
- *Shake It Up Baby!* Mix ingredients for the dressing right in the salad bowl, then layer the salad ingredients as directed. Cover tightly with plastic wrap. Use elastic bands around the edge of the bowl to keep the plastic wrap in place. Salad bowl must be tightly covered or you will be wearing your salad instead of eating it! At serving time, shake bowl to combine all the ingredients. Now that's exercising your options, and your body, too!

Mediterranean Kidney Bean Salad
(See recipe, page 96)

Mixed Greens with Mandarins, Berries and Pears
(See recipe, page 98)

Quinoa, Black Bean and Corn Salad
(See recipe, page 99)

Rainbow Tabbouleh Salad
(See recipe, page 101)

Raspberry Vinaigrette
(See recipe, page 102)

Red Cabbage Cole Slaw
Red cabbage dyes anything it touches purple. It's culinary magic—pour the hot dressing over the salad, and the cabbage will turn a brilliant magenta color!

1 medium head red cabbage, cored and thinly sliced (about 6 cups sliced)
2 medium carrots, peeled and grated
¾ cup chopped red onion
1 red or green pepper, seeded and chopped
2 cloves garlic (about 2 tsp minced)
¼ cup balsamic vinegar
¼ cup extra virgin olive oil
¼ cup granulated sugar or granular Splenda
2 tbsp minced fresh dillweed
½ tsp celery seed (optional)
Salt and freshly ground black pepper

1. Combine the cabbage, carrots, onion, red pepper, and garlic in a large mixing bowl.
2. In a 2-cup glass measure, combine the vinegar, oil, and sugar. Microwave, uncovered, on high for 45 seconds or until almost boiling. Pour the hot dressing over the vegetables and toss to mix well. Add the dillweed, celery seed (if using), salt, and pepper to taste; mix well.
3. Cover and refrigerate for at least 1 hour, or overnight, to blend the flavors. Adjust seasonings before serving.

Yield: 8 to 10 servings. Keeps for up to 1 week in the refrigerator.

154 calories per serving, 22.0 g carbohydrate, 3.9 g fiber, 3 g protein, 7.3 g fat (1.0 g saturated), 0 mg cholesterol, 52 mg sodium, 456 mg potassium, 1 mg iron, 77 mg calcium.
***Sweet Choice**—With Splenda, one serving contains 132 calories and 16.5 g carbohydrate.*

Chef's Secrets

- *It's a Slice:* To properly slice a cabbage, first peel off and discard any tough or dry outer leaves. Using a large sharp knife, cut the cabbage through the stem end into 4 pieces, then cut out and discard the hard white core attached at the base of each quarter. Cut each piece crosswise into very thin slices.
- *Processor Power:* You can also use your food processor (fitted with the slicing blade) to slice the cabbage; just cut the cabbage into wedges small enough to fit through the feed tube. Slice the cabbage wedges, using very light pressure on the pusher.
- *Quickie Slaw:* Substitute a bag of coleslaw mix or broccoli slaw (shredded broccoli stems) for the red cabbage.

Roasted Sweet Potato Salad
(See recipe, page 103)

Romaine, Avocado and Mango Salad with Citrus Dressing
(See recipe, page 104)

Tofu Antipasto
Debbie Jeremias likes to serve this as one of several salads for Shabbat. "It goes like crazy!"

    1 cup mushrooms, quartered
    2 stalks celery, sliced
    3 medium ripe tomatoes, diced
    1 red pepper, diced
    1 yellow pepper, diced
    1 orange pepper, diced
    2 green onions, sliced
    2 cloves garlic, thinly sliced

⅓–½ cup pitted black olives, halved
¾ lb firm tofu, diced (about 1-½ cups)
2 tbsp balsamic vinegar
2 tbsp olive oil (preferably extra virgin)
1 tsp dried oregano
1 tsp dried basil
Sea salt and freshly ground pepper, to taste

1. Combine all ingredients in a large bowl and mix well. If you have time, let mixture stand for 20 to 30 minutes to develop the flavor. (Can be made several hours in advance and refrigerated.)

Yield: 8 servings. Leftovers will keep for 2 or 3 days in the refrigerator.

140 calories per serving, 8.2 g fat (1.2 g saturated), 0 mg cholesterol, 8 g protein, 12 g carbohydrate, 73 mg sodium, 454 mg potassium, 6 mg iron, 3 g fiber, 116 mg calcium

Chef's Secret
- To lower calories and fat, use 1% silken extra-firm tofu. A 3-ounce (84 g) serving of tofu contains 35 calories and 1 g fat. Its texture is softer than regular firm tofu, but it works well in this recipe.

Turkish Eggplant Salad
(See recipe, page 106)

Wheat Berry Salad
(See recipe, page 107)

■ SIDE DISHES

Low-calorie side dishes can add a big fiber boost. Avoid potatoes; instead, heap on more vegetables or whole grains such as brown rice, whole-wheat bread, or kasha.

Barley Risotto with Portobello Mushrooms and Sun-Dried Tomatoes

Pearl barley makes a terrific substitute for Arborio rice in this creamy, non-traditional risotto—it's less expensive and has a lower glycemic index value, making this fiber-packed dish very "smart-carb." The portobello mushrooms and sun-dried tomatoes add a rich elegance to this humble grain. There will barely be any barley once they taste this!

½ cup (about 8 to 10) sun-dried tomatoes (if packed in oil, rinse well)
1 cup boiling water
4-½ cups vegetable or chicken broth
1-½ tbsp olive oil
½ red onion (about 1 cup chopped)
2 cups chopped portobello mushrooms
2 cloves garlic (about 2 tsp minced)
1-½ cups pearl barley, rinsed and drained
1 tsp minced fresh thyme or ½ tsp dried
2 tbsp minced fresh basil or 1 tsp dried
Salt and freshly ground black pepper

1. Combine the sun-dried tomatoes with boiling water in a small bowl. Let stand for 10 minutes to rehydrate. Drain, cut into bite-sized pieces, and set aside. (Scissors work well.) Heat the broth to simmering (either in the microwave or in a saucepan over medium-low heat), about 8 to 10 minutes.
2. Meanwhile, heat the oil in a large pot on medium high heat. Add the onion, mushrooms, and garlic; sauté for 5 minutes or until tender. If necessary, add

a little water to prevent sticking or burning. Stir in the barley and cook for 2 to 3 minutes or until lightly toasted, stirring to thoroughly coat the grains.

3. Reduce heat to low and slowly stir in ½ cup of hot broth. Cook and stir for about 2 minutes or until the broth evaporates. Add another ½ cup of broth and continue stirring until you can drag a spoon along the bottom of the pot and almost no liquid remains. Repeat twice more, adding ½ cup of broth each time and stirring constantly.

4. Pour in the remaining 2-½ cups of broth. Cover and simmer for 40 to 45 minutes, stirring occasionally, until the barley is tender. Add the sundried tomatoes, thyme, basil, salt, and pepper; mix well. Remove from the heat, cover, and let stand 5 minutes longer.

Yield: 12 servings of ½ cup each. Keeps for up to 3 days in the refrigerator; reheats well, especially in the microwave. Freezes well for up to 2 months.

133 calories per serving, 25.1 g carbohydrate, 5.1 g fiber, 4 g protein, 2.3 g fat (0.3 g saturated), 0 mg cholesterol, 224 mg sodium, 262 mg potassium, 1 mg iron, 24 mg calcium

Variations
- You can substitute up to 1 cup dry white wine for part of the broth.
- Instead of mushrooms, substitute 1 bunch asparagus, ends trimmed. Cut on the diagonal into 1-inch slices and lightly steam for 3 to 4 minutes before adding to the barley in Step 4. Frozen peas also make a great "green" option.

Basic Brown Rice
Brown rice has its bran layer intact. It's not polished like white rice, so it contains more nutrients, has a chewy texture and a nutty flavor. Short grain is stickier and chewier than long grain. Basmati brown rice has a mild flavor and is great for those who find regular brown rice too healthy-tasting!

2-¼ cups water, vegetable or chicken broth
1 cup long-grain brown rice, rinsed and drained

½ tsp salt

1 clove minced garlic, optional

½ tsp each basil, oregano, or thyme, optional

1. Place water or broth in a 2-quart heavy-bottomed saucepan. Cover and bring to a boil. Meanwhile, rinse rice; drain well. Add to boiling liquid along with desired seasonings. Bring back to a boil and simmer covered for 45 minutes. Remove from heat and let stand covered for 10 minutes, until liquid is absorbed. Fluff with a fork.

Yield: 6 3-cup servings. Reheats well. Do not freeze.

115 calories per ½ cup serving, 0.9 g fat (0.2 g saturated), 0 mg cholesterol, 3 g protein, 24 g carbohydrate, 199 mg sodium, 45 mg potassium, trace iron, 2 g fiber, 10 mg calcium

Variations

- *Brown Rice in Half the Time!* Rinse and drain rice. Combine with water and salt in a saucepan. Soak at room temperature for several hours or overnight. (I do this in the morning, then cook it at mealtime.) Bring rice to a boil, reduce heat and simmer tightly covered for just 22 minutes! Turn off heat and let rice stand covered for 10 minutes.
- *Oven Method:* Combine boiling liquid, rice, and desired seasonings in an ovenproof casserole. Cover tightly. Bake in a preheated 350°F oven for 50 to 60 minutes, until all liquid is absorbed.
- **Vegetable Un-Fried Rice:** Cook brown rice as directed. Prepare 2 to 3 cups of any of the following: bean sprouts, snow peas, chopped celery, green onions, red pepper, mushrooms, broccoli florets. Add 1 tbsp each of minced garlic and ginger to vegetables. Microwave covered on HIGH for 5 minutes, until tender-crisp. (No oil is needed, only a few drops of water to create steam.) Combine vegetables with cooked rice. Add 3 tbsp soy sauce, 2 to 3 tsp Oriental sesame oil, salt and pepper to taste.

- **Brown Rice Pilaf:** Cook brown rice as directed, using vegetable or chicken broth. Prepare 2 cups of any of the following vegetables: chopped onions, peppers, celery, carrots, mushrooms, broccoli, and/or cauliflower florets. Microwave covered on HIGH for 5 minutes. Add veggies to rice. Season with basil and thyme. Add salt and pepper to taste.
- *Chef's Cooking Secrets!* If cooked rice sticks to the bottom of the pot, place a heat diffuser or flame-tamer under the pot during cooking. If any liquid remains at the end of cooking, drain it off and place covered pot on low heat for a few minutes so that rice can dry out. If rice is too dry at the end of cooking, add a couple of spoonfuls of water, place pot on low heat and steam a few minutes longer.

Beans and Carrots Amandine

Full of fiber and flavor. Yellow beans can be substituted. Almonds are a terrific source of calcium.

1 tsp tub margarine, butter or olive oil
2 cloves garlic, crushed
¼ cup sliced almonds
2 cups green beans, cut in half crosswise
2 cups carrots, cut into matchsticks
½ cup water
¼ tsp salt
½ tsp dried basil (or 1 tbsp fresh basil)
Salt and pepper, to taste
2 tbsp grated Parmesan cheese, optional

1. Combine margarine and garlic in a 1 cup Pyrex measuring cup. Microwave uncovered on HIGH for 45 seconds. Stir in almonds. Microwave on HIGH for 3 to 4 minutes, until golden, stirring at half time. (Alternately, toast almonds with margarine and garlic in a nonstick skillet for 3 or 4 minutes.)

2. Combine green beans, carrots, water, and salt in a 2-quart microsafe casserole. Microwave covered on HIGH for 7 to 8 minutes, stirring at half time. Let stand covered for 2 or 3 minutes. Veggies should be tender-crisp. Drain well. Combine vegetables with seasonings and almonds. Sprinkle with Parmesan cheese if desired.

Yield: 4 servings. Reheats well in the microwave.

120 calories per serving, 5.8 g fat (0.2 g saturated), 0 mg cholesterol, 4 g protein, 15 g carbohydrate, 207 mg sodium, 403 mg potassium, 2 mg iron, 6 g fiber, 79 mg calcium

Broccoli, Mushroom and Pepper Sauté

This is great over pasta! Don't overcook broccoli. Heat destroys some of its protective antioxidants.

> 2 cups broccoli florets
> 4 cups cold water plus 1 tbsp vinegar
> 2 tsp olive oil
> 2 cloves garlic, crushed
> 2 cups mushrooms, sliced
> ½ cup red or yellow pepper, diced
> Salt and pepper, to taste
> 1 tbsp fresh basil, minced (or ½ tsp dried)

1. Soak broccoli in cold water and vinegar for 10 minutes. Drain and rinse well. Steam broccoli for 2 to 3 minutes (or microwave it). In a large nonstick skillet, heat oil. Add garlic, mushrooms and pepper; stir-fry for 2 minutes. Add broccoli and stir-fry 2 minutes more. Add seasonings and serve.

Yield: 4 to 6 servings.

54 calories per serving, 2.7 g fat (0.4 g saturated), 0 mg cholesterol, 3 g protein, 7 g carbohydrate, 22 mg sodium, 368 mg potassium, 1 mg iron, 3 g fiber, 44 mg calcium

Variations

- **Cauliflower, Mushroom and Pepper Sauté:** Substitute cauliflower florets in the previous recipe.
- **Quick Basil and Orange Broccoli:** Cover and microwave 3 cups cut-up broccoli on HIGH for 5 minutes. Add 2 tbsp orange juice, 1 tsp margarine or olive oil, salt, pepper, and a dash of basil. Yummy!

Bulgur with Almonds and Raisins

Bulgur is actually precooked cracked wheat so it doesn't require cooking, just soaking. While the bulgur soaks in water, take a soak in your bathtub and you'll both be ready at the same time.

1-½ cups medium bulgur
1-½ cups boiling water or vegetable broth
½ cup slivered almonds
2 tbsp extra virgin olive oil
3 tbsp lemon or orange juice (preferably fresh)
¼ cup chopped fresh basil or 1 tsp dried
½ cup raisins
1 tsp salt (or to taste)
¼ tsp freshly ground black pepper

1. Place the bulgur in a heat-resistant bowl and add boiling water or broth. Cover the bowl with a large plate and let stand for about 30 minutes or until the liquid is absorbed and the bulgur is tender.
2. Meanwhile, toast the almonds in a toaster oven for 5 to 7 minutes at 350°F or until golden and fragrant. (Or toast in a skillet on medium heat, stirring frequently, about 5 minutes.) Watch carefully to prevent the almonds from burning.
3. Stir the olive oil, lemon juice, basil, and raisins into the bulgur. Season with salt and pepper, and top with toasted almonds. Serve hot or at room temperature.

Yield: 6 servings. Keeps for up to 3 days in the refrigerator; reheats well. Freezes well for up to 2 months. Add the toasted almonds only at serving time.

253 calories per serving, 38.7 g carbohydrate, 8.1 g fiber, 7 g protein, 9.8 g fat (1.1 g saturated), 0 mg cholesterol, 395 mg sodium, 317 mg potassium, 2 mg iron, 45 mg calcium

Variations

- Instead of raisins, add dried cranberries, sliced dried apricots, or dried mango. Instead of almonds, substitute toasted walnuts, pecans, or pine nuts. Instead of bulgur, substitute 3 cups of cooked rice, millet, quinoa, or kasha.

Chef's Secrets

- *Love Me Tender:* Bulgur has a tender, chewy texture and makes a nice alternative to rice. Although this dish is best made with medium bulgur, you can use fine bulgur as well. If you use coarse bulgur, you will have to cook it first. Bulgur is delicious in pilafs, salads, meat, poultry, and vegetable dishes.

Company Stuffed Spuds

My friend Peter loves these! They're a favorite at his family's Passover Seder, or any time of year.

8 large baking potatoes (preferably Idaho)
4 green onions, trimmed and chopped
1 red pepper, chopped
1 tbsp olive oil
2 cloves garlic, crushed
½–¾ cup chicken or vegetable broth
2 tbsp minced fresh dill
1 tsp dried basil
Salt and pepper, to taste

1. Scrub potatoes well. Pierce skin in several places with a fork. Bake 400°F for 1 hour, until tender. Cool slightly. In a nonstick skillet, sauté onions and red pepper in oil until golden. Add garlic and cook 2 minutes longer. Add a little water if veggies start to stick or burn. Cut a slice off the top of each potato. Scoop out pulp, leaving a wall about ¼-inch thick. Mash potatoes. Add remaining ingredients; mix well. Mixture should be moist, but not mushy! Restuff skins. (Can be prepared in advance, covered and refrigerated.) Bake uncovered at 375°F for 25 minutes, until golden.

Yield: 8 servings. These reheat well or may be frozen.

243 calories per serving, 1.9 g fat (0.3 g saturated), 0 mg cholesterol, 5 g protein, 52 g carbohydrate, 28 mg sodium, 886 mg potassium, 3 mg iron, 5 g fiber, 32 mg calcium

Chef's Secret

- *Quicker Baked Potatoes:* Insert a metal skewer into each potato. Bake at 425°F for 30 to 40 minutes. Never bake potatoes wrapped in foil. They will steam and become soggy!

Couscous, Moroccan-Style

This delicious one-pot dish, with its blend of exotic Moroccan flavors, is a favorite of Shayla Goldstein of Toronto. It's great for busy families.

1-½ cups chicken broth (or a mixture of half orange juice and half water)
⅛ tsp ground cumin
⅛ tsp ground coriander
⅛ tsp ground ginger (optional)
1 cup whole-wheat couscous
2 green onions, finely chopped
⅓ cup dried cranberries or chopped dried apricots
¼ cup shelled pistachios or pine nuts

1. In a small saucepan over high heat, bring the broth, cumin, coriander, and ginger, if using, to a boil. Stir in the couscous, green onions, cranberries, and pistachios.
2. Remove the pan from the heat; cover and let stand for 5 minutes. Fluff with a fork and serve.

Yield: 4 servings. Recipe doubles or triples easily. Keeps for up to 3 days in the refrigerator; reheats well. Freezes well for up to 2 months.

190 calories per serving, 34.1 g carbohydrate, 5.2 g fiber, 6 g protein, 4.3 g fat (0.4 g saturated), 0 mg cholesterol, 187 mg sodium, 137 mg potassium, 2 mg iron, 30 mg calcium

Curry Roasted Cauliflower

Whenever my assistant Shelley Sefton makes this high fiber, high-flavor dish for family and friends, everyone asks when she's going to make it again. If making this for a crowd, double the recipe or make one of the variations. Shelley says that she can eat the whole thing by herself. So can I!

> 1 large cauliflower
> 1 red pepper, seeded and cut into long, narrow strips
> 2 tbsp olive oil
> 2 tsp curry powder
> ½ tsp salt (or to taste)
> ¼ cup sliced fresh chives or green onions, for garnish

1. Preheat the oven to 400°F. Line a large baking tray with parchment paper or sprayed foil.
2. Wash the cauliflower well and cut into large florets. Place in a large bowl along with the red pepper strips. Drizzle with oil and sprinkle with curry powder and salt; toss to mix. Spread in a single layer on the prepared baking tray. (If desired, the vegetables can be prepared a few hours in advance and set aside.)

3. Roast, uncovered, for 40 to 45 minutes until golden and crispy; halfway through the cooking process, stir the vegetables around. When roasted, some of the vegetables will be blackened around the edges—that's okay. Remove the vegetables from oven and sprinkle with chives. Serve immediately.

Yield: 4 to 6 servings. Leftovers, if any, are best served at room temperature. Don't freeze.

124 calories per serving, 13.6 g carbohydrate, 6.2 g fiber, 5 g protein, 7.2 g fat (1.0 g saturated), 0 mg cholesterol, 355 mg sodium, 724 mg potassium, 1 mg iron, 56 mg calcium

Variations

- **Rosemary Roasted Cauliflower:** Instead of curry powder, use 2 tsp dried rosemary and 2 to 3 cloves minced garlic.
- **Roasted Cauliflower Medley:** Add 1 to 2 cups of sliced mushrooms, sliced Japanese eggplant, and zucchini (don't peel). Baby carrots are also delicious. If you add more vegetables, you'll need 3 to 4 tbsp olive oil and 1 tbsp curry powder. If desired, add a little ground cumin and turmeric for extra flavor.

Chef's Secret

- *Leftovers?* Top with crumbled goat cheese and slivered sun-dried tomatoes. You can also add leftover roasted vegetables to an omelet, pasta, or soup.

Glazed Sweet Potatoes

Sweet potatoes are virtually fat-free and provide nearly half the daily recommended nutrient intake of vitamin C. Most important of all, they're delicious!

    2 onions, peeled and sliced
    4 sweet potatoes, peeled and cut in 2-inch chunks
    2 tsp olive oil or melted margarine
    2 tbsp maple syrup or honey

Salt and pepper, to taste
¼ tsp dried basil
¼ cup orange juice

1.   Preheat oven to 375°F. Spray a 2-quart covered Pyrex casserole with non-stick spray. Arrange onions in the bottom of the casserole; add sweet potatoes. Drizzle with olive oil and maple syrup. Sprinkle with seasonings. Drizzle orange juice over potatoes. Rub sweet potatoes well to coat them evenly with mixture. Cover and bake at 375°F for 45 minutes. Uncover and bake 15 minutes longer, stirring once or twice, until potatoes are tender and golden.

Yield: 6 servings. Reheats well, but do not freeze.

158 calories per serving, 1.9 g fat (0.3 g saturated), 0 mg cholesterol, 2 g protein, 34 g carbohydrate, 15 mg sodium, 278 mg potassium, <1 mg iron, 3 g fiber, 36 mg calcium

Time-Saving Secret!
- Microwave them covered on HIGH for 12 to 14 minutes, stirring once or twice. Potatoes will be partially cooked. Transfer casserole to a preheated 375°F oven. Bake uncovered 20 to 25 minutes, until tender, basting occasionally. If necessary, add a little more orange juice or water to casserole.

Great Grilled Vegetables
"Veg-out" at your next barbecue with this easy Mediterranean-style dish. When the weather is bad, you can roast the vegetables in a hot oven. This dish is a winner at any temperature.

1 large red onion, sliced in rings
3 bell peppers (red, orange, and/or yellow), cut in chunks
8 medium portobello mushrooms, halved
1 small eggplant, ends trimmed, sliced into ½-inch thick rounds
2 zucchini, sliced diagonally ½-inch thick

4 cloves garlic (about 4 tsp minced)

¼ cup extra virgin olive oil

¼ cup balsamic vinegar

2 tsp Kosher or sea salt

Freshly ground black pepper

¼ cup lightly packed chopped fresh basil or 2 tsp dried

1 tbsp chopped fresh oregano or 1 tsp dried

1 cup crumbled feta or goat cheese (optional)

1. In a large bowl, combine the onion, bell peppers, mushrooms, eggplant, and zucchini. Add the garlic, oil, balsamic vinegar, and salt and pepper to taste; mix well. Marinate for at least 30 minutes (or cover and refrigerate overnight).

2. Transfer the marinated vegetables to a perforated grilling basket, reserving any leftover marinade. (If you don't have a grilling basket, use heavy-duty foil that has been slashed in several places.) Grill over medium-high heat, stirring 2 or 3 times, for 18 to 20 minutes or until the vegetables are golden brown and tender-crisp.

3. Transfer the vegetables from the grill to a large serving platter. Add the reserved marinade, basil, and oregano; mix well. Top with cheese, if using, at serving time.

Yield: 8 servings. Keeps for up to 2 to 3 days in the refrigerator. Don't freeze.

134 calories per serving, 14.6 g carbohydrate, 4.5 g fiber, 4 g protein, 7.4 g fat (1.0 g saturated), 0 mg cholesterol, 331 mg sodium, 738 mg potassium, 1 mg iron, 33 mg calcium

Oven-Roasted Vegetables

-   Instead of grilling vegetables, spread them in a single layer on a large baking tray that has been lined with sprayed foil. Roast, uncovered, and stir occasionally, for 20 to 25 minutes at 425°F, or until golden brown and tender-crisp.

Variations
- Omit the eggplant and cheese and add 2 Belgian endives, trimmed and halved lengthwise. Add 1 tbsp honey along with oil, vinegar, and seasonings. Serve with grilled chicken breasts or salmon on a bed of salad greens.

Chef's Secrets
- *Herb Magic:* If using dried herbs, add them at the beginning of the cooking process. Thyme or rosemary also make flavorful seasonings.
- *Leftovers?* Use in wraps, or brighten up any pasta, rice, or grain dish with these colorful vegetables.

Homemade Baked Beans

Full of flavor, fiber, iron and calcium, yet low in fat. These are a nutritional bargain. No time to make beans? For a great shortcut, add 2 to 3 tablespoons maple syrup to a can of baked beans. Just heat and eat!

1 lb (454 g) white beans (e.g., navy)
6 cups water
2 onions, chopped
¼ cup sugar (white or brown)
⅓ cup molasses
2 tbsp red wine vinegar
1-¾–2 cups tomato juice
1 tsp dry mustard
¼ tsp cayenne (to taste)
½ tsp black pepper
Salt, to taste

1. Soak beans overnight; rinse and drain well. Cook in 6 cups unsalted water for 45 to 60 minutes, until tender. Reserve cooking water from beans; set aside. Preheat oven to 275°F. In an ovenproof dish, combine drained beans with remaining ingredients plus 1 cup of reserved cooking water. Bake covered until tender, about 5 hours. Add more water if needed to prevent mixture from drying out.

Yield: 10 servings. These taste even better a day or two later!

215 calories per serving, 0.8 g fat (0.2 g saturated), 0 mg cholesterol, 10 g protein, 44 g carbohydrate, 160 mg sodium, 674 mg potassium, 4 mg iron, 7 g fiber, 105 mg calcium

Honey-Glazed Carrots

This is a honey of a dish because you don't need to peel or cut the carrots, which is so a-peeling! These glazed carrots are perfect for the Jewish High Holidays, Passover, or any time of year.

> 2 lb (1 kg) baby carrots
> 2 tbsp extra virgin olive oil
> 2 tbsp lemon juice (preferably fresh)
> 2 tbsp honey
> 2 tbsp apricot or mango preserves (preferably low-sugar or all-fruit)
> Salt and freshly ground black pepper
> ½ tsp dried thyme
> ¼ cup chopped fresh parsley or dillweed, for garnish

1. Place the carrots in a medium saucepan and add enough water to cover by 1 inch; bring to a boil. Reduce heat to low and simmer, covered, for 12 to 15 minutes or until tender. Drain well and return the carrots to the saucepan.
2. Add the oil, lemon juice, honey, jam, salt, pepper, and thyme. Cook for 2 or 3 minutes longer, stirring to prevent sticking, until the carrots are nicely glazed. Garnish with parsley and serve.

Yield: 6 servings. Recipe doubles or triples easily. Keeps for up to 3 days in the refrigerator; reheats well. Don't freeze.

127 calories per serving, 21 g carbohydrate, 2.9 g fiber, 1 g protein, 4.9 g fat (0.7 g saturated), 0 mg cholesterol, 120 mg sodium, 383 mg potassium, 2 mg iron, 54 mg calcium

Variations

- **Maple Balsamic Carrots:** Replace the lemon juice and honey with balsamic vinegar and maple syrup.
- Instead of using baby carrots, substitute 3 bags (10 oz/300 g each) of grated carrots: the carrots will cook in about 10 minutes. Instead of lemon juice and apricot jam, use orange juice and orange marmalade.

Chef's Secrets

- *Baby Bonus:* Baby carrots are a terrific time-saver because they don't require peeling. They are actually regular carrots that have been cut by a machine into mini carrots. It takes 1 medium carrot to make 4 or 5 baby carrots. Bagged baby carrots are not fresh if they have a white tinge on the outside.
- *Carrot Cuisine:* Carrots are also delicious in soups, salads, stews, casseroles, grain dishes, side dishes, cakes, muffins, and quick breads. Enjoy them raw, roasted, steamed or stir-fried, or add them raw to salads. Very versatile.

Microwaved Oriental Broccoli

Broccoli is an Italian word that means "little arms." Your guests are sure to welcome this nutritious, delicious dish with open arms.

1 clove garlic (about 1 tsp minced)
1 small slice peeled fresh ginger (about 1 tbsp)
2 tbsp orange juice (preferably fresh)
1 tbsp soy sauce (low-sodium or regular)
2 tsp honey
1 tsp Asian (toasted) sesame oil
1 large bunch broccoli (about 1-½ lb/750 g)
½ cup seeded and finely chopped red pepper, for garnish
¼ cup toasted slivered almonds, for garnish

1. In a food processor fitted with the steel blade, process the garlic and ginger until finely minced. Add the orange juice, soy sauce, honey, and sesame oil; process for 6 to 8 seconds or until blended. (If desired, the sauce can be prepared in advance and refrigerated for 1 to 2 days.)
2. Rinse the broccoli thoroughly in cold water, shaking off any excess. Trim the woody ends and cut the broccoli into florets. Slice the thick parts of the stems into 1-inch pieces. Place the broccoli in a large microwaveable bowl. Cover and microwave on high for about 5 minutes or until tender-crisp and bright green. Don't overcook. Drain well.
3. Drizzle the sauce over the broccoli and mix gently. Transfer to a serving dish and garnish with the red pepper and toasted almonds.

Yield: 4 servings. Recipe doubles or triples easily. Serve hot or at room temperature. Don't freeze.

123 calories per serving, 16.8 g carbohydrate, 5.7 g fiber, 6 g protein, 5.2 g fat (0.5 g saturated), 0 mg cholesterol, 184 mg sodium, 593 mg potassium, 2 mg iron, 92 mg calcium

Variations

- This sauce also tastes marvelous over asparagus, cauliflower, or green beans. Try it with broccoli raab, which is similar to broccoli but has fewer florets and more stems.
- Substitute ¼ cup bottled Asian salad dressing or sauce instead of making your own.

Chef's Secrets

- *Time It Right:* Microwave broccoli, covered, on high, allowing 4 to 5 minutes per pound. Microwave ovens vary in wattage, so some experimentation might be necessary.
- *Nuts to You!* To toast almonds, microwave, uncovered, on high for 2 minutes.
- *Steam Power:* Instead of microwaving broccoli, cook it in a vegetable steamer for 5 minutes.

- *Microwave Magic:* When you microwave broccoli, there's no need to add water. The residual moisture from washing the broccoli is sufficient to create steam for cooking. Use parchment paper that has been rinsed under cold water to cover the cooking dish—wetting the paper makes it flexible so you can mold it easily around the dish.

Millet Pilaf

Millet is not just for the birds! This easy-to-digest grain is found in health food stores. It is high in protein, complex carbohydrates, phosphorus, potassium, iron, calcium, and B vitamins. Millet triples in volume, so use a large pan. Pre-toasting eliminates bitterness and prevents mushy millet!

1 tbsp olive or canola oil
2 medium onions, chopped
1 stalk celery, chopped
1 red pepper, chopped
1 green pepper, chopped
2 cloves garlic, minced
1 cup mushrooms, sliced
1 cup millet
2-¼ cups water, chicken or vegetable broth
½ tsp dried basil
½ tsp dried thyme
Salt and freshly ground pepper, to taste
¼ cup chopped fresh parsley

1. Heat oil in a nonstick skillet. Add vegetables and sauté on medium-high heat until golden, about 5 to 7 minutes. If necessary, add a couple of tablespoons of water or broth if veggies begin to stick. (Or microwave veggies covered on HIGH for 5 minutes, omitting oil.)

2. Rinse and drain millet thoroughly. Place in a large heavy-bottomed fry-pan and toast it on medium heat for about 5 minutes, stirring constantly to prevent burning. It's ready when it gives off a toasty aroma similar to popcorn. Remove from heat and add broth slowly to prevent spattering. Add remaining ingredients except parsley. Cover and simmer for 20 to 25 minutes. Add parsley and let stand covered for 5 to 10 minutes. Fluff with a fork.

Yield: 6 servings. Reheats well. Leftovers keep 3 or 4 days in the fridge. (I usually don't have any!)

173 calories per serving, 3.9 g fat (0.6 g saturated), 0 mg cholesterol, 5 g protein, 31 g carbohydrate, 13 mg sodium, 230 mg potassium, 2 mg iron, 4 g fiber, 27 mg calcium

Chef's Secrets
- If you cook veggies without oil, 1 serving contains 153 calories and 1.6 g fat (0.3 g saturated).
- Millet can be stored in a tightly sealed container in the refrigerator or freezer for up to 4 months. Don't store it at room temperature for more than a couple of weeks, particularly in hot weather. If millet smells musty, throw it out.
- *Variations*: For added crunch, add 2 tablespoons toasted sesame seeds, pine nuts or slivered almonds to cooked millet mixture.
- **Milletburgers:** Process leftover Millet Pilaf on the steel knife of your processor with a little soy, tamari, or teriyaki sauce until mixture holds together. (Millet should be somewhat moist and sticky for best results.) Combine with beaten egg (or egg whites) and some bread crumbs or matzo meal. Press firmly into patties. Brown on both sides in a little canola or olive oil in a nonstick skillet.

Minted Peas with Red Peppers

Green peas are more nutritious than green beans! They contain vitamins A and C and are high in fiber.

    10 oz pkg (300 g) frozen green peas
    2 tsp tub margarine or olive oil
    4 green onions (white part only), chopped
    1 red pepper, chopped
    1–2 tbsp fresh mint, minced
    Salt and freshly ground pepper, to taste
    1 tbsp fresh lime or lemon juice

1. Bring a saucepan of water to a boil. Add peas and simmer 3 to 4 minutes, until tender-crisp. Drain and rinse well under cold water to stop the cooking process. Set aside. Melt margarine in a nonstick skillet. Add onions and red pepper. Sauté for 4 or 5 minutes, until softened. Add peas and mint. Cook for 1 to 2 minutes, just until heated through. Add seasonings and lime juice. Serve immediately.

Yield: 3 to 4 servings.

104 calories per serving, 2.8 g fat (0.5 g saturated), 0 mg cholesterol, 5 g protein, 16 g carbohydrate, 99 mg sodium, 217 mg potassium, 2 mg iron, 5 g fiber, 29 mg calcium

Variation

- **Rice Pea-laf with Peppers:** Prepare Minted Peas with Red Peppers as directed above. Combine with 3 cups of cooked brown basmati rice. Add salt and pepper to taste.

Oven-Roasted Asparagus

This fiber-packed dish is a snap to prepare. Roasting concentrates the flavor of the asparagus and the tips will get very crispy. Warning—this is addictive.

 1-½ lb (750 g) asparagus spears
 2 tbsp extra virgin olive oil
 2 tbsp lemon juice (preferably fresh) or balsamic vinegar
 2 cloves garlic (about 2 tsp minced)
 Sea salt or Kosher salt

1. Preheat the oven to 425°F. Line a large baking tray with foil; spray with cooking spray.
2. Soak asparagus thoroughly in cold water; drain well. Bend asparagus and snap off the tough ends at the point where they break off naturally. Place in a single layer on the prepared baking sheet. Drizzle with olive oil, lemon juice, and garlic. Roll the asparagus to coat all sides.
3. Roast, uncovered, in the lower third of the oven for 12 to 15 minutes or until the spears are tender-crisp and lightly browned. Using tongs, turn the asparagus once or twice during roasting for even browning. Transfer to a platter, lightly sprinkle with salt, and serve.

Yield: 4 to 6 servings. Recipe doubles or triples easily. Serve hot or at room temperature. Don't freeze.

102 calories per serving, 7.7 g carbohydrate, 3.2 g fiber, 4 g protein, 7.4 g fat (1.1 g saturated), 0 mg cholesterol, 22 mg sodium, 370 mg potassium, 1 mg iron, 40 mg calcium

Variations

- **Cæsar's Spears:** Omit the oil, lemon juice, and garlic, and instead coat the asparagus with ¼ cup low-calorie Cæsar dressing. Sprinkle with 2 tbsp sesame seeds and 2 tbsp grated Parmesan cheese. Roast as directed above. Romans, seize your spears!

- **Grilled Asparagus:** Preheat the grill. Prepare the asparagus as directed in Step 2. Transfer to the hot grill, laying spears crosswise to prevent them from falling through the cracks in the grate, or place in a grill basket. Grill over medium-high heat for 7 to 8 minutes or until the spears are lightly browned and somewhat crispy.
- **Herb-Roasted Asparagus:** Add 1 tsp minced fresh rosemary, thyme, tarragon, or dried Italian seasoning to the olive oil, lemon juice, and garlic. Roast or grill.

Chef's Secrets

- *Juicy Secrets:* The zest from citrus fruits such as lemons adds a fresh citrus flavor to asparagus without discoloring it. So instead of adding lemon juice to asparagus, add finely grated lemon zest. Lemon aid, without the juice!

Potato and Carrot Purée

Such a lovely pale, orange color. This yummy purée is full of flavor and vitamins, yet low in fat.

> 4 large potatoes (preferably Yukon Gold)
> 3 large carrots
> 3 cloves garlic, peeled
> Salted water for cooking potatoes
> ¾ cup skim milk (or use rice or soy milk)
> Salt and freshly ground pepper, to taste
> ½ tsp dried basil (or 1 tbsp fresh)
> 1 tsp tub margarine or olive oil, optional

1. Peel potatoes and carrots and cut them into chunks. Place in a saucepan along with garlic. Cover with water and bring to a boil. Reduce heat and simmer covered about 20 minutes, until tender. Drain well. Return potatoes, carrots, and garlic to the saucepan. Dry over medium heat for about a minute to evaporate any water. Meanwhile, heat milk (about 45 seconds on HIGH in the microwave).

2.   Mash potatoes, carrots, and garlic with a potato masher, or put them through a food mill. (Do not use a processor or your potatoes will be like glue!) Add hot milk and beat until light and creamy. Add salt, pepper, basil, and margarine and mix well. Serve immediately.

Yield: 6 servings. These reheat beautifully in the microwave.

106 calories per serving, 0.2 g fat (0.1 g saturated), <1 mg cholesterol, 3 g protein, 24 g carbohydrate, 42 mg sodium, 432 mg potassium, <1 mg iron, 3 g fiber, 61 mg calcium

Variations

- *Pareve Version:* Reserve ½ to ¾ cup of the cooking water from potato/carrot mixture. Add hot liquid to mashed potato mixture in Step 2.
- **Two Potato Purée:** Substitute 1 sweet potato for the carrots. Blend in 1 tablespoon light cream cheese.

Rainbow Rice Pilaf

Pretty as a picture! Colorful and vitamin-packed, this easy side dish also makes a fabulous filling for Vegetarian Stuffed Peppers (page 170). Fresh vegetables can be used instead of frozen.

2 cups vegetable broth
1 cup long-grain or basmati rice, rinsed and drained
2 tsp olive oil
1 large onion, finely chopped
2 cloves garlic, crushed
½ cups green pepper, finely chopped
½ cup red pepper, finely chopped
1 cup zucchini, finely chopped
1-½ cups frozen mixed vegetables, thawed
Salt and pepper, to taste

1.	In a medium saucepan, bring broth to a boil. Add drained rice to saucepan, cover and simmer on low heat for 20 minutes. Remove from heat and let stand covered for 10 minutes. Meanwhile, heat oil in a nonstick skillet. Add onion and sauté for 5 minutes. Add garlic, peppers, and zucchini. Sauté 4 or 5 minutes longer, until tender-crisp. If necessary, add a little broth or water to prevent sticking. Stir in mixed vegetables. Cover and let stand for 5 minutes to heat through. Combine veggie mixture with rice. Season to taste. Fluff with a fork.

Yield: 6 servings. Leftovers keep 2 days in the fridge and reheat well. Freezing is not recommended.

193 calories per serving, 2.3 g fat (0.3 g saturated), 0 mg cholesterol, 6 g protein, 39 g carbohydrate, 355 mg sodium, 238 mg potassium, 2 mg iron, 4 g fiber, 36 mg calcium

Refried Black Beans

My friend Kathy Guttman, of Toronto, who loves food with an extra spicy kick, shared this tasty dish with me. If you do too, add even more cumin, chili powder, and/or hot sauce than what's called for in this recipe. These refried black beans makes for a zesty side dish with grilled salmon, beef, or chicken.

1 tsp olive oil
1 small onion, chopped
1 can (19 oz/540 ml) black beans, drained (do not rinse)
2 cloves garlic (about 2 tsp minced)
¼ tsp ground cumin (or to taste)
½ tsp chili powder (or to taste)
Salt and freshly ground black pepper
1 small tomato, chopped
¼ cup minced fresh cilantro
4 to 6 drops hot sauce (optional)

1. Heat oil in a large nonstick skillet over medium heat. Add the onion and
    sauté for 3 to 4 minutes or until softened. Stir in the black beans, garlic,
    cumin, chili powder, salt, and pepper; continue sautéing for 3 to 4 min-
    utes to blend the flavors. Add the tomato, cilantro, and hot sauce, if using.
2. Remove the pan from the heat and, using a potato masher, immersion
    blender, or fork, mash until the mixture is somewhat creamy, but with
    some beans still whole or partially mashed. Serve warm.

Yield: About 2 cups (6 servings of ⅓ cup). Keeps for up to 3 days in the
refrigerator. Reheats well in the microwave. Don't freeze.

*64 calories per serving, 13.7 g carbohydrate, 4.5 g fiber, 4 g protein, 0.9 g fat (0.1 g sat-
urated), 0 mg cholesterol, 351 mg sodium, 302 mg potassium, 1 mg iron, 34 mg calcium*

Chef's Secrets

- *Using Your Bean:* For maximum flavor, drain the black beans but don't
  rinse them.
- *Bean Cuisine:* Black beans are so versatile—use them in appetizers,
  spreads, soups, sauces, stews, chili, burritos, or salads.

Nutrition Notes

- *Lean Beans:* Most canned refried black beans are made with lard—this
  homemade version is much healthier.
- *Salt Alert!* Organic brands of canned beans are lower in sodium than
  regular brands.
- *Black Beans Are Best*: Black beans are easier to digest than most beans,
  making them a top choice when it comes to legumes. They're packed
  with antioxidants and fiber and are high in protein. Eating black beans
  helps to lower cholesterol, stabilizes blood sugar, and reduces your cancer
  risk. Black beans also have a lower glycemic index (GI 42), and they're
  high in folate, an essential nutrient for pregnant women.

Roasted Root Vegetables

Let's get back to our roots! Thanks to Hester Springer and my mom for this great recipe.

2 beets, peeled and sliced
2–3 potatoes, peeled and cut in wedges
2 large onions, quartered
2 sweet potatoes, peeled and cut in chunks
3–4 carrots, peeled and cut in chunks
2 parsnips, peeled and cut in chunks
1 medium turnip, peeled
2 tbsp olive oil
2 tbsp balsamic or red wine vinegar
3–4 cloves garlic, crushed
Salt and pepper, to taste
1 tsp dried basil or thyme (or 1 tbsp fresh)

1. Preheat oven to 400°F. Mix vegetables together with oil, vinegar, garlic, and seasonings. Place in a single layer on a sprayed nonstick baking pan. Bake uncovered for 45 to 55 minutes, until tender and browned, stirring occasionally. Serve immediately.

Yield: 8 servings.

160 calories per serving, 3.7 g fat (0.5 g saturated), 0 mg cholesterol, 3 g protein, 30 g carbohydrate, 157 mg sodium, 580 mg potassium, 1 mg iron, 5 g fiber, 55 mg calcium

Variations

• My mom uses beets but omits the sweet potatoes and parsnips. My friend Hester omits the beets but uses sweet potatoes, parsnips, and turnips. You can use whichever vegetables you like!

- **Roasted Fennel with Onions:** Use 2 large onions and 2 fennel bulbs, cut in wedges. Mix together with 2 cloves crushed garlic, 1 tbsp olive oil and 2 tbsp balsamic vinegar. Add salt and pepper to taste. Cook as directed for Roasted Root Vegetables (page 221). Makes 4 servings.

Sesame Green Beans

For a colorful presentation, use a combination of green and yellow wax beans. Cut the red peppers into strips about the same size as the beans. Prepare all the ingredients in advance and cook just before serving. It will be ready to eat in minutes.

¼ cup water, or chicken or vegetable broth
2 tbsp soy sauce (low-sodium or regular)
1 tsp granulated sugar or granular Splenda
1 tbsp canola oil
2 green onions, trimmed and chopped
3 to 4 cloves garlic (about 3 to 4 tsp minced)
2 tsp peeled and minced fresh ginger
1 lb (500 g) green beans, trimmed
1 red pepper, seeded and cut into long, narrow strips
Salt and freshly ground black pepper
2 tsp Asian (toasted) sesame oil
2 tbsp sesame seeds

1. In a small bowl, combine the water, soy sauce, and sugar; set aside.
2. Heat the oil in a wok or large nonstick skillet on medium high heat. Add the green onions, garlic, and ginger, and stir-fry for 1 minute. Add the green beans and red pepper strips; stir to coat well. Cook for 1 minute longer.
3. Add the reserved soy sauce mixture and bring to a boil. Cover, reduce heat to low, and simmer for 4 to 5 minutes or until tender-crisp. Season with salt and pepper to taste and toss with the sesame oil.
4. Transfer the cooked beans to a platter. Sprinkle with sesame seeds and serve immediately.

Yield: 4 servings. Can be reheated briefly in the microwave. Don't freeze.

142 calories per serving, 15.4 g carbohydrate, 4.9 g fiber, 4 g protein, 8.4 g fat (0.7 g saturated), 0 mg cholesterol, 544 mg sodium, 284 mg potassium, 2 mg iron, 81 mg calcium

Simple and Good Ratatouille
(See recipe, page 165)

Simply Sautéed Greens

    1 tbsp olive oil
    1 red pepper, chopped
    2–3 cloves garlic, crushed
    2 lb greens, well-trimmed, washed and drained

1.   In a wok or large skillet, sauté red pepper and garlic in oil for 2 minutes. Chop tender leaves into 1-inch pieces and add gradually to the pan. Reduce heat to medium, cover and cook until tender, stirring occasionally. (Beet greens and spinach take 2 to 3 minutes, Swiss chard and broccoli raab take 3 to 4 minutes, and kale takes 5 to 8 minutes.) Add a few tablespoons of water if mixture becomes dry. Season with salt and pepper. Remove greens from the pan with a slotted spoon.

Yield: 4 servings.

114 calories per serving (for kale), 4.4 g fat (0.6 saturated), 0 mg cholesterol, 5 g protein, 15 g carbohydrate, 54 mg sodium, 579 mg potassium, 2 mg iron, 3 g fiber, 176 mg calcium

Simply Steamed Asparagus

1-½ lb (750 g) asparagus, trimmed and cut into 2-inch slices
Salt and pepper, to taste
1 tsp fresh thyme leaves (or ¼ tsp dried)
3 tbsp fresh lemon, lime, or orange juice
1 tsp tub margarine (or 2 tsp light tub margarine)

1. Soak asparagus in cold water; drain well. Steam for 3 to 4 minutes. Immediately transfer to a bowl of ice water to stop the cooking process. (To microwave asparagus, place it in an oval casserole and microwave covered on HIGH for 6 to 7 minutes, until tender-crisp. Let stand covered for 3 minutes.) Season with salt, pepper, and thyme. Sprinkle with juice. Add margarine and mix well. At serving time, reheat for 2 or 3 minutes on HIGH in the microwave.

Yield: 4 to 6 servings. Do not freeze.

50 calories per serving, 1.5 g fat (0.3 g saturated), 0 mg cholesterol, 4 g protein, 8 g carbohydrate, 26 mg sodium, 269 mg potassium, 1 mg iron, 3 g fiber, 35 mg calcium

Variation
- **Asparagus Vinaigrette:** Steam asparagus as directed. Omit lemon juice and margarine. Sprinkle asparagus with salt, pepper, and thyme. Toss with nonfat or low-fat Italian salad dressing.

Spring Mix Vegetable Medley

This colorful vegetable medley is delicious as a side dish or served over pasta. The recipe can be halved easily, but I always make a big batch because it's so versatile. Leftovers make a delicious snack right from the refrigerator.

2 medium onions, halved and sliced
2 red peppers, seeded and cut in strips

2 cups sliced mushrooms

1 lb (500 g) asparagus (tough ends trimmed), cut diagonally into 2-inch pieces

1 large zucchini or yellow squash, unpeeled and cut into strips

3 to 4 cloves garlic (about 3 to 4 tsp minced)

3 tbsp extra virgin olive oil

3 tbsp lemon juice (preferably fresh) or rice vinegar

2 tsp sea salt or Kosher salt

Freshly ground black pepper

2 tbsp minced fresh dillweed (plus additional for garnish)

1 tbsp minced fresh thyme or 1 tsp dried

½ cup sesame seeds

1. Place the prepared vegetables in a large bowl. Add the garlic, olive oil, lemon juice, salt, pepper, dillweed, and thyme; mix well. (If desired, the vegetables can be prepared in advance up to this point and refrigerated, covered, for several hours or overnight.)

2. Preheat the oven to 425°F. Line a large baking tray with foil and spray with cooking spray.

3. Spread the vegetables in a single layer on the prepared baking tray and sprinkle with sesame seeds. Roast, uncovered, for 15 to 18 minutes or until golden brown and tender-crisp, stirring once or twice. Transfer to a serving platter and garnish with additional dillweed. Serve hot or at room temperature.

Yield: 6 servings. Keeps for up to 3 days in the refrigerator. To reheat, bake uncovered at 375°F for 10 to 12 minutes. Don't freeze.

122 calories per serving, 13.2 g carbohydrate, 3.5 g fiber, 3 g protein, 7.4 g fat (1.1 g saturated), 0 mg cholesterol, 440 mg sodium, 452 mg potassium, 7 mg iron, 40 mg calcium

Variations

- Substitute trimmed green beans for asparagus. This recipe is also tasty with small cauliflower florets. For a spicy kick, add 1 tsp red pepper flakes or smoked paprika to the seasoning mixture in Step 1.
- This versatile combination makes a delicious topping for chicken, fish, pasta, or grains. To turn this into a vegetarian main dish, make Spaghetti Squash with Roasted Vegetables (page 295).

Squished Squash

Nutrient-packed, rich in beta-carotene and folic acid, this dish is potassi-yummy!

2 acorn squash or 1 butternut squash
1–2 tbsp tub margarine or olive oil
Salt and pepper, to taste
¼ tsp each of ground cinnamon and nutmeg

1. Preheat oven to 375°F. Cut squash in half crosswise. Place cut-side down on a sprayed nonstick baking pan. Bake uncovered until tender, about 50 to 60 minutes.
2. Cool slightly, then scoop out and discard seeds and stringy pulp from squash. Scoop out the flesh from squash into a bowl and mash together with margarine/olive oil and seasonings. Reheat before serving.

Yield: 4 servings. Do not freeze.

103 calories per serving, 3.1 g fat (0.6 g saturated), 0 mg cholesterol, 2 g protein, 20 g carbohydrate, 30 mg sodium, 601 mg potassium, 1 mg iron, 6 g fiber, 65 mg calcium

Chef's Secrets

- To microwave squash, pierce in several places with a sharp knife. Place on microsafe paper towels and microwave on HIGH, allowing 5 to 7 minutes per pound. Turn squash over halfway through cooking. Total cooking time will be 12 to 14 minutes. Complete as directed in Step 2.

- *Squash, anyone?* Winter varieties include acorn, buttercup, butternut, Hubbard, pumpkin, spaghetti, and turban squash. They do not need refrigeration. Store at room temperature for about a month.

Sweet Potato "Fries"

Everyone loves sweet potato fries. These make a delicious and much healthier alternative to traditional French fries made from regular potatoes. If you like, sprinkle sweet potato fries with your favorite vinegar at serving time. Yam good!

3 medium sweet potatoes, well-scrubbed or peeled
2 tbsp extra virgin olive oil
1 tsp Kosher or sea salt
Freshly ground black pepper
1 tsp sweet paprika
1 tsp garlic powder

1. Preheat the oven to 425°F. Line a large baking sheet with foil—this makes for easier clean-up. Place the baking sheet in the lower third of the oven to heat up.
2. Meanwhile, cut the sweet potatoes into ¼-inch strips or wedges. Combine in a large bowl with oil, salt, pepper, paprika, and garlic powder. Using your hands, toss the sweet potatoes in the oil and spices to coat well on all sides.
3. When the oven is fully heated, spread out the sweet potatoes onto the hot baking sheet so that they will brown well.
4. Bake in the lower third of the oven for 20 minutes. Turn the sweet potato pieces over with a spatula and continue baking until brown and crispy, about 20 to 25 minutes longer. Serve immediately.

Yield: 4 servings. Freezes well for up to 2 months. Reheats well.

180 calories per serving, 27.3 g carbohydrate, 3.8 g fiber, 2 g protein, 7.2 g fat (1.0 g saturated), 0 mg cholesterol, 361 mg sodium, 358 mg potassium, 5 mg iron, 41 mg calcium

Variations

- Season with salt and pepper; omit the paprika and garlic powder. Sprinkle with ground cinnamon and nutmeg, or sprinkle with seasoning salt, chili powder, Cajun spices, basil, curry powder, or any spices you like.

Chef's Secrets

- *Frozen Assets:* Sweet potatoes freeze well, unlike white potatoes. If you do freeze, there's no need to thaw when reheating: just spread the frozen "fries" on a foil-lined baking sheet and bake, uncovered, at 400°F for about 10 to 12 minutes.
- *Confused?* Sweet potatoes are not yams, although they are often marketed that way. Sweet potatoes usually have an orange flesh, but can also be yellow, white, or even purple. The darker the flesh, the moister and sweeter they are. Sweet potatoes with dark orange flesh have more vitamin A than those with lighter color flesh. The skin can be different colors, including red-orange, brown, and purple. Yams are bigger, usually have white flesh, thick, dark-brown skin and tend to be bland, floury, and starchy; they are never sweet.

Vegetable Platter Primavera

2 cups broccoli florets
2 cups cauliflower florets
1 cup carrots, sliced on the bias
1 cup sliced zucchini or yellow squash
4 green onions (white part only), sliced
½ cup red pepper, diced
1 tbsp olive oil (or melted margarine)
2 tbsp lemon juice
1 tbsp water
Salt and pepper, to taste
2 tbsp minced fresh basil and/or dill

1.   Soak broccoli, cauliflower, and carrots in cold water for 10 minutes. Drain well but do not dry. Arrange broccoli and cauliflower florets in a ring around the outer edge of a large microwave-safe plate. Make an inner ring of carrots, then of zucchini. Place green onions and red pepper in the center. Combine olive oil, lemon juice, and water; drizzle over vegetables. Cover with an inverted Pyrex pie plate or a damp paper towel.

2.   Microwave covered on HIGH for 6 to 8 minutes, until tender-crisp. Let stand covered for 2 minutes. Season with salt, pepper and herbs. Serve immediately.

Yield: 6 servings. Do not freeze.

62 calories per serving, 2.7 g fat (0.4 g saturated), 0 mg cholesterol, 3 g protein, 9 g carbohydrate, 111 mg sodium, 351 mg potassium, <1 mg iron, 4 g fiber, 45 mg calcium

Variation

- **Vegetable Platter with Cheese Sauce:** Cook vegetables as directed, omitting oil. Melt 1 teaspoon tub margarine for 20 seconds on HIGH in the microwave. Stir in 2 tablespoons flour. Gradually whisk in 1 cup skim milk. Microwave uncovered on HIGH until steaming hot, about 2 minutes, whisking at half time. Blend in ½ cup grated low-fat cheddar cheese. Add salt, pepper, and ½ teaspoon dried mustard. Stir well. Drizzle sauce over hot vegetables.

Vegetarian Harvest Oven Stir-Fry

So colorful, so healthy!

1 medium eggplant, unpeeled
1 red, 1 yellow, and 1 green pepper
1 medium Spanish onion (about 2 cups)
2 medium zucchini, unpeeled
2 cups sliced mushrooms (try shiitake or portobello)
4 cloves garlic, crushed

1 tbsp olive oil

2 tbsp balsamic or red wine vinegar

Salt and pepper, to taste

2 tbsp fresh chopped rosemary or basil (or 1 tsp dried)

1. Preheat oven to 425°F. Cut eggplant, peppers, onion, and zucchini into narrow strips. Combine all ingredients in a large bowl. (May be prepared in advance, covered, and refrigerated for 3 or 4 hours.) Spread in a thin layer on a large foil-lined baking sheet that has been sprayed with nonstick spray.
2. Place baking sheet on top rack of oven. Bake uncovered for 25 to 30 minutes, until tender-crisp and lightly browned, stirring once or twice.

Yield: 6 servings. This dish reheats well either in the microwave or conventional oven. Veggies become soggy if frozen.

99 calories per serving, 3 g fat (0.4 g saturated), 0 mg cholesterol, 3 g protein, 18 g carbohydrate, 8 mg sodium, 532 mg potassium, 2 mg iron, 5 g fiber, 55 mg calcium

Variation

- **Rozie's Vegetable Medley:** Prepare vegetable mixture as directed in Step 1 of Vegetarian Harvest Oven Stir-Fry, omitting eggplant. Peel 2 sweet potatoes and cut them into chunks. Add 2 or 3 carrots, thickly sliced (or 2 cups baby carrots). Microwave sweet potatoes and carrots covered on HIGH for 4 to 5 minutes, until tender-crisp. Combine with remaining ingredients and mix well. If desired, add 1 cup of snow peas and/or canned baby corn, rinsed and drained. Either cook veggies in the oven as described above, or place them in a sprayed grill basket or perforated wok designed for the BBQ. Grill until nicely browned and tender-crisp, about 20 to 30 minutes, stirring occasionally.

■ FISH DISHES

While fish contains no fiber, it's a low-fat, high-quality protein. Mix it with high fiber vegetables or grains, and you have a nutrient-packed meal.

Asian Tuna Salad
(See recipe, page 132)

Creamy Salmon Filling in Toast Cups
(See recipe, page 133)

Fast Fish Salad
(See recipe, page 134)

Grilled Tuna with Mango Salad
The recipe for this impressive dish comes from the cookbook *Cooking Kindness*, compiled by my friend Gloria Guttman of Toronto. You can prepare the salad in advance and grill the tuna just before serving.

> 1 large mango, peeled, pitted, and cut into ¼-inch wide strips
> ¾ cup chopped red onion
> ½ cup chopped red pepper
> 3 tbsp chopped fresh cilantro
> 2 tbsp rice vinegar
> 2 tbsp extra virgin olive oil
> Salt and freshly ground black pepper
> 4 yellowfin tuna steaks, about 1-inch thick (5 to 6 oz/150 to 180 g each)
> 1 tbsp canola oil

1. *Mango Salad:* Combine the mango, onion, red pepper, cilantro, rice vinegar, and olive oil in a medium bowl; season with salt and pepper. (Can be made several hours in advance and refrigerated.)

2. *Grilled Tuna:* Set the grill to medium-high heat (or preheat the broiler). Lightly brush both sides of the tuna steaks with oil. Grill or broil just until the tuna is opaque in the center, about 3 to 4 minutes per side. Don't overcook.

3. Divide the mango salad among 4 plates and top with the grilled tuna.

Yield: 4 servings. Keeps for up to 1 to 2 days in the refrigerator. Don't freeze.

298 calories per serving, 13 g carbohydrate, 1.7 g fiber, 34 g protein, 12.1 g fat (1.6 g saturated), 64 mg cholesterol, 55 mg sodium, 796 mg potassium, 1 mg iron, 36 mg calcium

Variations
- Instead of grilled tuna, top Mango Salad with Asian Tuna Salad (page 132).

Pecan-Crusted Tilapia
You'll go nuts over this dish once you try it! The crusty coating is a terrific source of fiber.

> 4 tilapia fillets (6 oz/175 g each)
> ¼ cup dried breadcrumbs (whole-grain is best)
> ¼ cup wheat bran, oat bran, or whole-wheat flour
> ¼ cup finely chopped pecans
> ½ tsp salt (or to taste)
> ¼ tsp freshly ground black pepper
> ¼ tsp garlic powder
> ½ tsp paprika
> 1 tbsp olive or canola oil
> 1 egg plus 1 tbsp water
> 4 lemon wedges, for garnish

1. Preheat the oven to 425°F. Line a baking sheet with foil and spray with cooking spray.

2. Cut each fillet in half, lengthwise, making two long pieces. Cut the thicker piece in half crosswise (tilapia fillets have a thicker side and a

thinner side). You should end up with three long pieces that are all the same thickness—this helps the fish to cook evenly.

3. Combine the breadcrumbs, bran, pecans, salt, pepper, garlic powder, paprika, and oil in a shallow dish and set aside. Whisk the egg and water together in a pie plate. Dip the fish first in the egg wash, making sure all sides are coated. Quickly dredge both sides of the dipped fish in the breadcrumb mixture.

4. Arrange the breadcrumb-coated fish in a single layer on the prepared baking sheet. (You can prepare the fish in advance up to this point and refrigerate for 3 to 4 hours.)

5. Bake, uncovered, for 10 minutes or until golden. (There's no need to turn the fish over while baking.) Serve hot, garnished with lemon wedges.

Yield: 4 to 6 servings. Keeps for up to 2 days in the refrigerator; reheats well. Don't freeze: if frozen, the coating won't be crispy.

300 calories per serving, 8.6 g carbohydrate, 2.7 g fiber, 38 g protein, 13.4 g fat (2.3 g saturated), 138 mg cholesterol, 449 mg sodium, 612 mg potassium, 2 mg iron, 43 mg calcium

Variations

- Any firm-fleshed fish fillets will work—try it with sole, snapper, flounder, or dore/pickerel.
- Substitute almonds, hazelnuts, or any nuts you like instead of pecans.
- Instead of dipping fish fillets in beaten egg, dip them in low-calorie honey mustard or Italian salad dressing, then in the crumb mixture.

Chef's Secrets

- *What's in Store:* Tilapia is a farm-raised fish that is low in fat and has a mild, delicious flavor. It is white-fleshed, fine textured, and often tinged with pink.
- *Cook It Right:* Here's another technique to prevent overcooking. Cut each fillet in half lengthwise, making two long pieces. Coat each piece with the breadcrumb mixture as directed in Step 2. Thinner pieces take 10 minutes to bake and thicker pieces take 2 to 3 minutes longer.

- *Pan-tastic!* Don't add the oil to the breadcrumb mixture. Instead of baking, pan-fry the fish in a nonstick skillet in 1 to 2 tbsp oil on medium-high heat for 2 to 3 minutes per side. Drain on paper towels.

Pepper-Crusted Tuna

This looks absolutely fabulous served on a bed of mixed salad greens drizzled with your favorite salad dressing. It's definitely upper crust!

6 yellowfin tuna steaks, about 1-inch thick (5 to 6 oz/150 to 180 g each)
2 tbsp canola oil
¾ cup sesame seeds
3 tbsp coarsely cracked black peppercorns

1. Preheat the grill or broiler. Lightly brush both sides of the tuna steaks with oil. Combine the sesame seeds with the peppercorns. Press the sesame seed mixture onto both sides of the tuna. (Can be prepared up to 1 hour in advance and refrigerated.)
2. Grill or broil the tuna just until it is opaque in the center, about 3 to 4 minutes per side. Don't overcook. Slice diagonally across the grain into thin slices and serve immediately.

Yield: 6 servings. Keeps for up to 1 to 2 days in the refrigerator. Don't freeze.

307 calories per serving, 4.7 g carbohydrate, 2.6 g fiber, 37 g protein, 14.5 g fat (0.7 g saturated), 64 mg cholesterol, 87 mg sodium, 667 mg potassium, 2 mg iron, 93 mg calcium

Chef's Secrets

- *Skillet or Grill It?* Instead of grilling the tuna, use a heavy skillet and sear in hot oil for 2 to 3 minutes per side or until the outer edges are just cooked but the center is still rare.
- *Company's Coming!* Artfully arrange the slices of tuna on top of Apricot Hoisin Spinach Salad (page 83) or use the pepper-crusted tuna slices in Grilled Tuna with Mango Salad (page 231).

Quick Pickled Salmon
(See recipe, page 135)

Salmon Patties
A lighter version of a family favorite! Leftover cooked fish can be used.

    1 small onion
    ½ stalk celery
    1 tbsp fresh dill (or ½ tsp dried)
    2 slices whole-wheat bread
    7-½ oz can (213 g) salmon, drained (use bones—they contain calcium!)
    1 egg plus 2 egg whites (or 2 eggs)
    1 tsp Worcestershire sauce
    1 tsp lemon juice
    Freshly ground pepper, to taste
    1 tbsp canola oil (for frying)

1. In the processor, mince onion, celery, and dill. Moisten bread under cold running water; squeeze out excess moisture. Add bread to processor; process until finely ground. Add remaining ingredients except oil. Process with quick on/offs, until mixed. Mixture will be quite moist but will hold together. In a large nonstick skillet, heat oil on medium-high heat. Drop mixture by tablespoons into skillet. Flatten slightly with the back of the spoon. Cook on medium heat until brown, about 3 or 4 minutes per side.

Yield: 8 patties. Reheats and/or freezes well.

88 calories per patty, 4.1 g fat (0.8 g saturated), 37 mg cholesterol, 8 g protein, 4 g carbohydrate, 210 mg sodium, 145 mg potassium, <1 mg iron, <1 g fiber, 79 mg calcium

Variations

- **Tuna Patties:** Substitute a 6-½ oz can (184 g) water-packed tuna, drained. Each patty contains 77 calories, 2.9 g fat (0.49 saturated), 33 mg cholesterol, 159 mg sodium, and 120 mg potassium.
- **Salmon or Tuna Muffins:** Prepare mixture. Bake in sprayed muffin tins 25 minutes, until golden.
- *Leftovers?* Patties are great in sandwiches the next day. Tuck into a pita pocket, or serve on rye, kimmel, or black bread. Top with lettuce, tomatoes, and cucumber slices. Garnish with sprouts.
- **Salmon or Tuna Loaf:** Prepare mixture for Salmon Patties, but triple the recipe, using only 1 egg (or 2 whites) for each can of salmon or tuna. Omit oil. Spray a 9- by 5-inch loaf pan with nonstick spray. Sprinkle with corn flake crumbs. Pour in fish mixture. Bake at 350°F for about 1 hour. Makes 6 to 8 servings. Leftovers are great cold the next day in sandwiches.

Tuna Caponata

(See recipe, page 136)

Tuna, Rice and Broccoli Kugel

Excellent for family or friends. It's perfect for a buffet and wonderful for brunch. Cheese and milk are excellent sources of calcium Broccoli is a good source of calcium and contains beta carotene.

2 cups water
Salt, to taste
1 cup long-grain rice
3 cups broccoli, coarsely chopped
1 onion, chopped
6-½ oz can (184 g) tuna, drained and flaked
2 tomatoes, diced
3 eggs plus 2 egg whites
1 cup skim milk

1 cup nonfat or low-fat yogurt
¼ tsp each of basil and oregano
1 cup grated low-fat mozzarella or Swiss cheese
3 tbsp grated Parmesan cheese

1. In a medium saucepan, bring water and a dash of salt to a boil. Add rice, cover and simmer for 20 minutes. (Alternately, microwave rice, water, and salt covered on HIGH for 6 to 7 minutes. Reduce power to 50% [MEDIUM]; microwave 10 to 12 minutes longer, until water is absorbed.) Let rice stand covered for 10 minutes using either cooking method.

2. Microwave broccoli and onion covered on HIGH for 4 minutes. Let stand covered for 2 minutes. Broccoli should be tender-crisp. Combine with remaining ingredients except Parmesan cheese and mix well. Spread evenly in a lightly greased or sprayed 7- by 11-inch Pyrex casserole. Sprinkle with Parmesan cheese. (Can be prepared in advance up to this point, covered, and refrigerated for several hours or overnight.) Bake in a preheated 350°F for 45 minutes, until golden brown.

Yield: 8 servings. Reheats well and/or may be frozen.

212 calories per serving, 3.4 g fat (1.3 g saturated), 89 mg cholesterol, 16 g protein, 29 g carbohydrate, 222 mg sodium, 427 mg potassium, 2 mg iron, 2 g fiber, 171 mg calcium

*   Use water-packed tuna, not oil-packed. You can use 2 cans of tuna for more protein.
*   Egg substitute can be used instead of eggs for those with cholesterol problems.
*   **Salmon, Rice and Broccoli Casserole:** Substitute salmon for tuna. (Green beans can replace the broccoli if you like, but then you have to change the name of the recipe!)

■ CHICKEN AND TURKEY

Once you remove the skin and fat, poultry is a lean protein that complements whole grains and vegetables.

Asian Chicken and Noodle Salad
(See recipe, page 138)

Chicken Breasts with Colored Peppers
Simply delicious! This recipe is a winner with my students.

Vegetables:
1 tsp olive oil
1 onion, sliced
1 green, 1 red, and 1 yellow pepper, sliced
2 large cloves garlic, crushed
2–3 tbsp water (as needed)
Salt and pepper, to taste
½ tsp dried basil (or 1 tbsp fresh, minced)
½ tsp dried thyme

Chicken:
4 skinless, boneless chicken breasts, trimmed of fat (about 1 lb/500 g)
Freshly ground pepper
2 tsp additional olive oil
2 green onions, minced
2 tbsp flour
½ cup chicken broth
½ cup dry white wine
1 tsp Dijon mustard (to taste)

1. *Vegetables:* Heat 1 teaspoon olive oil in a large nonstick skillet or wok. Add onion, peppers, and garlic. Sauté on medium heat until tender, about 5 minutes, adding a little water if vegetables begin to stick. (Or microwave the vegetables covered on HIGH for 5 minutes, omitting water.) Sprinkle with salt, pepper, basil, and thyme. Remove vegetables from skillet.

2. *Chicken:* Cut chicken breasts into strips or leave them whole. Sprinkle with pepper. Heat 2 teaspoons olive oil in wok. Stir-fry chicken breasts over medium-high heat for 2 to 3 minutes, until they turn white. Add green onions and cook 1 minute longer. Sprinkle flour over chicken. Cook about a minute longer to lightly brown the flour, scraping up any browned bits. Add broth, wine, and mustard. Stir until mixture comes to a boil. Reduce heat and simmer uncovered for 3 or 4 minutes, basting chicken occasionally. Stir in vegetables. Cook 2 to 3 minutes longer, until vegetables are hot. Adjust seasonings to taste.

Yield: 4 servings. This dish reheats well. If frozen, peppers may develop a slightly bitter taste.

251 calories per serving, 6.7 g fat (1.4 g saturated), 73 mg cholesterol, 30 g protein, 13 g carbohydrate, 119 mg sodium, 438 mg potassium, 2 mg iron, 2 g fiber, 48 mg calcium

Variations
- Serve on a bed of basmati rice or with boiled new potatoes.
- **Chicken Breasts with Mushrooms:** Use 2 cups sliced mushrooms instead of peppers. Freezes and reheats well.
- *Passover Version:* Substitute potato starch instead of flour. Substitute 1 tbsp of fresh lemon juice for mustard.

Chicken Fajitas

This easy, nutrition-packed dish is a fun way for a family to enjoy a meal together. It gives everyone a chance to be creative, adding the ingredients that they like. Let the good times roll!

4 boneless, skinless chicken breasts, cut into thin strips (about 1-½ lb/750 g)
Salt and freshly ground black pepper
2 cloves garlic (about 2 tsp minced)
1 tsp ground cumin
Juice of 1 lime (about 2 tbsp)
2 tbsp olive oil
1 large onion, thinly sliced
1 green and 1 red pepper, seeded and cut into strips
1 jalapeno chili pepper, seeded and cut into strips
6 10-inch flour tortillas (preferably whole-wheat), warmed

Additional Fillings:
2 cups shredded romaine lettuce
1 cup chunky salsa (bottled or homemade)
Optional: Refried Black Beans (page 219), guacamole, chopped tomatoes, cilantro

1. Rinse the chicken well and trim the excess fat. Place chicken in a medium bowl. Season it with salt, pepper, garlic, and cumin. Add the lime juice and 1 tbsp of the olive oil; mix well. Cover and marinate for 1 hour (or for up to 2 days in the refrigerator).
2. Heat the remaining 1 tbsp oil in a large nonstick skillet over medium high heat. Add the onion and peppers and sauté until tender, about 6 to 8 minutes. Transfer to a plate and set aside.
3. Pour the marinade from the chicken into the skillet and heat over medium high heat. (No need to wash the skillet first.) Add the chicken strips and sauté in the marinade until lightly browned, about 3 to 4 minutes. Using a slotted spoon, transfer the chicken to a plate.

4. *Assembly:* Spoon the chicken onto the warm tortillas, leaving a 1-inch border on the bottom and the sides. Top with the sautéed vegetables and desired fillings. Fold in the sides and the bottom of the tortilla, and roll up tightly into a cylinder. Serve immediately.

Yield: 6 servings. Recipe doubles or triples easily. Chicken freezes well for up to 3 months; reheats well. The vegetables will get soggy if frozen, then thawed.

401 calories per serving, 46.1 g carbohydrate, 4.1 g fiber, 25 g protein, 12.5 g fat (2.6 g saturated), 49 mg cholesterol, 718 mg sodium, 435 mg potassium, 4 mg iron, 131 mg calcium

Variation

- Instead of chicken, substitute thinly sliced lean beef such as London broil or extra-firm tofu.

Chicken Mango Salad with Peanut Dressing

(See recipe, page 140)

Chicken with Bulgur and Mushrooms

Easy, tasty, and nutritious! Rice can be substituted for the bulgur.

3 lb (1.4 kg) chicken, cut in pieces
3 onions, sliced
2 cups mushrooms, sliced
1 cup bulgur, rinsed and well-drained
2 cloves garlic, minced
Salt (optional)
Freshly ground pepper, to taste
1 tsp dried basil
2 cups vegetarian tomato sauce
¾ cup water

1. Wash chicken and remove skin. Trim off excess visible fat. Place onions, mushrooms, and bulgur in the bottom of a lightly greased casserole. Arrange chicken pieces on top. Rub chicken with garlic and seasonings. Combine sauce and water; pour over chicken and bulgur. Bake covered at 350°F for 1-¼ hours, or until chicken is tender and most of liquid is absorbed. Adjust seasonings to taste.

Yield: 6 servings. Reheats and/or freezes well.

330 calories per serving, 10 g fat (2.3 g saturated), 72 mg cholesterol, 29 g protein, 33 g carbohydrate, 516 mg sodium, 851 mg potassium, 3 mg iron, 7 g fiber, 60 mg calcium

Chef's Secrets
- If desired, chicken wings can be set aside and frozen. When you have enough saved up, make chicken soup!
- Serve with steamed zucchini and carrots seasoned with salt, pepper and dill.

Curried Chicken, Red Pepper and Mango Salad
(See recipe, page 141)

Glazed Apricot-Mustard Chicken Breasts with Rosemary
Mouth-watering! Dijon mustard is high in sodium, so no additional salt is needed.

6 single chicken breasts (with bone)
¼ cup Dijon mustard
¼ cup apricot jam
1 tbsp honey
1 tsp olive oil
2 tsp fresh rosemary (or 1 tsp dried)
Freshly ground pepper and paprika, to taste
Fresh rosemary, to garnish
14 oz can (398 ml) water-packed apricots, drained

1. Line a 10- by 15-inch baking sheet with foil; spray with nonstick spray. Remove skin from chicken. Trim off excess fat. In a small bowl, combine mustard, jam, honey, oil, and 2 tsp rosemary. Mix well. Rub chicken with mustard glaze, reserving any leftover glaze. Arrange chicken bone-side down on baking sheet. Sprinkle lightly with pepper and paprika. (Can be prepared in advance up to this point, covered and refrigerated for up to 24 hours.)

2. Preheat oven to 350°F. Bake chicken uncovered on middle rack for 45 minutes, brushing it with reserved glaze during last 15 minutes of cooking. When done, juices will run clear and chicken will be glazed and golden. Do not overcook or chicken will be dry. Arrange chicken on a serving platter. Garnish with rosemary. Arrange drained apricots attractively around chicken.

Yield: 6 servings. Freezes and/or reheats well. Recipe can be multiplied for a large crowd.

246 calories per serving, 4.9 g fat (1 g saturated), 73 mg cholesterol, 28 g protein, 23 g carbohydrate, 331 mg sodium, 437 mg potassium, 2 mg iron, 2 g fiber, 50 mg calcium

Variations
- Chicken legs and thighs can be used instead of breasts with the bone. Remove skin and fat; prepare as directed above. If using boneless breasts, bake 20 to 25 minutes at 400°F.
- Pineapple jam or orange marmalade can replace apricot jam. Dill or thyme can replace rosemary.
- Serve with Rainbow Rice Pilaf (page 218) and steamed asparagus.

High-Fiber Turkey Stuffing

1–2 tbsp olive oil

2 onions, chopped

3 stalks celery, chopped

2 cups mushrooms, sliced

3 carrots, grated

10 slices of rye or multi-grain bread

2 apples, cored, peeled, and chopped

Salt and pepper, to taste

2 tbsp fresh dill, chopped

2 tbsp fresh basil, chopped (or 1 tsp dried)

1 tbsp fresh thyme (or 1 tsp dried)

½–¾ cup chicken broth

1. Heat oil in a large, nonstick skillet. Sauté onions and celery until golden. Add mushrooms and carrots. Cook 5 minutes longer; remove from heat. Cut bread into cubes and add to skillet with remaining ingredients. Mix well. You will have enough for a 10- to 12-pound turkey. (Stuffing can be prepared up to 24 hours in advance and refrigerated, but don't add broth until just before cooking.) Remove excess fat from turkey neck and cavity. Stuff turkey loosely. Fold neck skin over and attach it with a skewer to the turkey. Cook turkey as per recipe directions, allowing 25 to 30 minutes per pound.

Yield: 10 servings. Reheats well. Freezing not recommended.

132 calories per serving, 2.6 g fat (0.7 g saturated), 0 mg cholesterol, 4 g protein, 24 g carbohydrate, 245 mg sodium, 182 mg potassium, 2 mg iron, 3 g fiber, 43 mg calcium

Variations

- **Passover Matzo Stuffing:** Substitute 6 pieces soaked, drained matzo for the bread.

- **Skinnier Stuffing:** Bake stuffing separately in a covered greased casserole at 325°F for 1 hour.
- **Stuffin' Muffins:** Bake stuffing in sprayed muffin tins at 350°F for 25 minutes, until crispy.

Hoisin Chicken and Broccoli Stir-Fry

Hoy-sinful! Hoisin sauce, also known as Chinese ketchup, is a thick, reddish-brown sauce with a sweet and spicy taste. It is made from a mixture of soybeans, garlic, chili peppers, and spices. This is delicious over cooked soba noodles (Japanese buckwheat noodles) or rice.

½ cup hoisin sauce
2 tbsp orange marmalade or apricot jam (preferably low-sugar or all-fruit)
2 tbsp lemon juice (preferably fresh)
1 lb (500 g) boneless, skinless single chicken breasts, cut into thin strips
2 tbsp canola oil
2 tsp minced garlic
2 tsp minced fresh ginger
1 red onion, thinly sliced
1 red pepper, thinly sliced
2 cups broccoli florets
2 cups mushrooms, sliced
2 cups bean sprouts
2 tsp cornstarch dissolved in
2 tbsp cold water or chicken broth

1. Combine the hoisin sauce, marmalade, and lemon juice in a large glass bowl; mix well.
2. Rinse the chicken well and pat dry. Trim the excess fat. Add the chicken and marinate for 30 minutes at room temperature (or refrigerate for up to 2 days). Drain the chicken, reserving marinade.

3.   Heat 1 tbsp oil on medium high heat in a large nonstick wok. Add the drained chicken, garlic, and ginger. Stir-fry for 2 to 3 minutes or until the chicken is no longer pink. Remove from the wok.

4.   Heat remaining oil. Stir-fry the onion, red pepper, broccoli, mushrooms, and bean sprouts on high heat for 2 minutes. Add the chicken, reserved marinade, and cornstarch mixture. Stir-fry 1 to 2 minutes longer or until bubbly and thickened. This is best served immediately.

Yield: 4 servings. Leftovers can be reheated in the microwave or a wok, but won't be as crunchy. Don't freeze.

361 calories per serving, 35.8 g carbohydrate, 4.7 g fiber, 32 g protein, 11.2 g fat (1.5 g saturated), 68 mg cholesterol, 590 mg sodium, 680 mg potassium, 3 mg iron, 64 mg calcium

Variations
- Substitute lean boneless beef or firm tofu, cut into strips, for the chicken breasts.
- Add 2 cups sliced water chestnuts or bamboo shoots to the wok along with reserved marinade.
- Garnish with ½ cup toasted cashews or slivered almonds.

Chef's Secrets
- *It's a Keeper:* Bottled hoisin sauce can be refrigerated for at least a year.
- *Saucy Secret:* Hoisin sauce adds body to stir-fries, so less cornstarch is needed to thicken the sauce.

Mushroom Turkey Loaf

This moist and flavorful loaf is made with dried shiitake mushrooms instead of breadcrumbs. It's packed with fiber and is an excellent source of iron. Although you can make half the recipe for a small family, I prefer to freeze the extra loaf for another day. Cook once, eat twice!

2 cups dried shiitake mushrooms
2 medium onions, cut in chunks

3 to 4 cloves garlic (3 to 4 tsp minced)

2 lb (1 kg) lean ground turkey

1 large egg plus 2 egg whites (or 2 large eggs)

⅓ cup hoisin, barbecue, or duck sauce

¾ tsp salt (or to taste)

½ tsp freshly ground black pepper

1 tsp dried basil

1 tsp dried oregano

1. Preheat the oven to 350°F. Line a baking sheet with foil and spray with cooking spray.
2. In a food processor fitted with the steel blade, process the dried mushrooms until finely ground, about 45 to 60 seconds. Transfer the ground mushrooms to a large mixing bowl.
3. Add the onions and garlic to the food processor and process with several quick on/off pulses, until minced. Transfer to the bowl with the mushrooms and add the ground turkey, egg, egg whites, hoisin sauce, and seasonings; mix lightly to combine.
4. Divide and shape the mixture into two loaves on the prepared baking sheet, wetting your hands for easier handling. (If desired, the turkey-vegetable mixture can be prepared in advance up to this point, covered and refrigerated overnight.)
5. Bake, uncovered, for 1 hour. Slice and serve.

Yield: 2 loaves (8 servings). Keeps for up to 2 days in the refrigerator; reheats well. Freezes well for up to 3 months.

341 calories per serving, 26.8 g carbohydrate, 5.4 g fiber, 32 g protein, 11.4 g fat (2.9 g saturated), 117 mg cholesterol, 551 mg sodium, 350 mg potassium, 8 mg iron, 50 mg calcium

Chef's Secrets

- *Switching A-Ground:* Instead of turkey, use extra-lean ground beef, veal, or chicken.

- *Mushroom Magic:* Substitute ground dried mushrooms for matzo meal or breadcrumbs in recipes—it adds flavor and moisture, especially to ground turkey, which can be bland because of its low fat content. One cup of dried shiitake mushrooms yields ½ cup when ground. Make an extra batch or two and store it in a cool dry place, or freeze it.

New-Fashioned Cabbage Rolls in Cranberry Sauce

Lean minced chicken or turkey replaces fatty ground beef, and cranberry sauce adds fabulous flavor to the sauce. You can also add a grated apple and a handful of raisins to the sauce.

Cranberry Sauce:
1 medium cabbage (about 3 lb/1.4 kg)
14 oz can (398 ml) jellied cranberry sauce
2 cups tomato sauce (preferably low-sodium)
1 cup water
⅓ cup brown or white sugar (to taste)
¼ tsp cinnamon
2 tbsp lemon juice (to taste)

Cabbage Rolls:
1-½ lb (750 g) ground chicken or turkey breast (remove skin and fat if grinding it yourself)
2 egg whites (or 1 egg)
4 green onions, minced
2 cloves garlic, minced
1 small carrot, grated
½ cup oatmeal, matzo meal, or bread crumbs
½ tsp salt
¼ tsp pepper

½ tsp dried basil
½ cup uncooked rice
½ cup water
3–4 tbsp ketchup

1. Remove 16 to 18 large leaves from cabbage. (Refer to Cabbage Without Damage! on page 250) Trim away the tough ribs; set aside. In a large pot, combine cranberry sauce, tomato sauce, water, sugar, cinnamon, and lemon juice. Bring to a boil, stirring to break up cranberry sauce. Cut up leftover cabbage and add to the sauce. While sauce is simmering, prepare the cabbage rolls.
2. Combine ground poultry with remaining ingredients and mix lightly. Place a large spoonful of filling on each cabbage leaf. Roll up, folding in ends. Place cabbage rolls seam-side down in the pot of sauce. If sauce doesn't cover cabbage, add a little water. Cover and simmer slowly for 1-½ to 2 hours, basting occasionally, until cabbage is tender.

Yield: 16 cabbage rolls. These reheat and/or freeze well.

177 calories per cabbage roll, 1.7 g fat (0.4 g saturated), 24 mg cholesterol, 11 g protein, 30 g carbohydrate, 168 mg sodium, 343 mg potassium, 1 mg iron, 3 g fiber, 48 mg calcium

Variations

- **Passover Cabbage Rolls or Meatballs in Cranberry Sauce:** Use white sugar instead of brown sugar in the sauce. Use matzo meal instead of oatmeal or bread crumbs in the chicken mixture. (You can even use matzo farfel; it will look like rice!) If making meatballs, omit cabbage and shape chicken mixture into small balls. Simmer meatballs for 1 to 1-½ hours, until tender.
- **Vegetarian Cabbage Rolls:** Refer to recipe (page 168).
- The sauce from Secret Ingredient Sweet and Sour Meatballs (page 268) can also be used for cabbage rolls.

Cabbage Without Damage!

- Large leaves are best for stuffing. Remove the core of cabbage with a sharp knife.
- *Freezer Method:* Place whole cabbage in a plastic bag in the freezer 2 days before. Remove cabbage from freezer the night before. Thaw overnight at room temperature. In the morning, the wilted leaves will separate easily.
- *Boiling Method:* Place the whole cabbage in a large pot of boiling water and simmer for 10 minutes, or until leaves are softened. When cool enough to handle, separate leaves.
- *Microwave Method:* Rinse cabbage but do not dry. Microwave covered on HIGH for 8 to 10 minutes, until outer leaves are pliable. Let stand covered for 3 or 4 minutes. Separate leaves. If cabbage is not flexible when you remove the last few leaves, microwave it 1 or 2 minutes longer.
- To roll cabbage leaves more easily, pare the thick rib portion with a sharp paring knife.

No-Fry Almond Schnitzel

You'll go nuts for these crispy, crunchy chicken breasts. The coating is healthy because of the good fat in the almonds and sesame seeds.

1 cup Special K cereal (⅓ cup when coarsely crushed)
⅓ cup wheat germ
¼ cup almonds
3 tbsp sesame seeds
½ tsp salt (or to taste)
½ tsp freshly ground black pepper
½ tsp garlic powder
½ tsp dried basil
½ tsp paprika
2 egg whites (or 1 large egg)
4 boneless, skinless single chicken breasts (1-½ lb/750 g)

1. Preheat the oven to 400°F. Line a baking sheet with parchment paper or foil sprayed with cooking spray.
2. In a food processor fitted with the steel blade, combine the cereal, wheat germ, almonds, sesame seeds, and seasonings; process for 15 to 20 seconds to make coarse crumbs. Transfer to a plate.
3. In a pie plate, lightly whisk the egg whites; set aside.
4. Rinse the chicken well and pat dry with paper towels. Trim the excess fat. Dip the chicken breasts first in the egg whites, then dredge both sides in the crumb mixture to thoroughly coat. Arrange the chicken in a single layer on the prepared baking sheet. (If desired, the chicken can be prepared in advance up to this point, covered, and refrigerated overnight.)
5. Bake, uncovered, for 20 to 25 minutes or until crisp and golden, turning chicken over after 10 minutes.

Yield: 4 servings. Recipe doubles or triples easily. Keeps for up to 3 days in the refrigerator; reheats well. Freezes well for up to 4 months.

346 calories per serving, 13.3 g carbohydrate, 3.1 g fiber, 44 g protein, 12.7 g fat (1.6 g saturated), 94 mg cholesterol, 472 mg sodium, 497 mg potassium, 5 mg iron, 70 mg calcium

Variation

- **Almond-Crusted Chicken Fingers.** Cut each chicken breast into 4 or 5 long strips. Coat as directed. Bake for 10 minutes, then flip and bake 6 to 8 minutes longer.

Chef's Secrets

- *Be Prepared:* Make several batches of the crumb mixture and store in re-sealable plastic bags in your refrigerator or freezer for up to 6 months.
- *Nut Allergies?* Omit the almonds and increase the amount of Special K cereal to 1-¾ cups.
- *GI Go!* Special K cereal has a lower glycemic index value than corn flakes, making it a healthier choice as a crispy coating.

Nutty-Baked Chicken

The inspiration for this crispy, high fiber dish comes from Natasha Goldberg of Chicago. She likes to use a mixture of nuts, so choose whatever kind you like. You'll go nuts when you taste this!

1 whole chicken (3-½ lb/1.6 kg), cut into pieces
Salt and freshly ground black pepper
2 tbsp light mayonnaise
1 tbsp Dijon mustard
¾ cup finely chopped nuts (almonds, walnuts, pecans, filberts, and/or
　　peanuts)
¾ cup wheat or oat bran
1 tbsp garlic powder
1 tbsp onion powder

1. Preheat the oven to 375°F. Line a large baking sheet with foil and spray with cooking spray.
2. Rinse the chicken well and pat dry with paper towels. Trim the excess fat and remove the skin. Season the chicken with salt and pepper to taste.
3. In a small bowl, combine the mayonnaise and mustard. Combine the nuts, wheat bran, garlic powder, and onion powder in a re-sealable plastic bag. Lightly brush the seasoned chicken pieces with the mayonnaise mixture, then place in the bag, one or two pieces at a time, and shake to thoroughly coat with the nut mixture. Transfer the coated chicken pieces to the prepared baking sheet, arranging them in a single layer.
4. Bake the chicken, uncovered, for about 1-¼ hours or until the coating is crispy and golden. Juices should run clear when the chicken is pierced with a fork.

Yield: 6 servings. Keeps for up to 3 days in the refrigerator; reheats well. Freezes well for up to 4 months. Don't cover when reheating or the chicken coating won't be crisp.

339 calories per serving (without skin), 9.3 g carbohydrate, 4.8 g fiber, 32 g protein, 20.4 g fat (3.3. g saturated), 92 mg cholesterol, 191 mg sodium, 426 mg potassium, 3 mg iron, 40 mg calcium

"Nut"-rition Notes

- Although nuts are high in fat and calories, they contain mostly unsaturated fat that helps protect your heart. Nuts are cholesterol-free and provide good sources of protein, phosphorus, zinc, and magnesium, along with vitamin E and selenium.
- *Go Nuts!* Different nuts have different benefits, so enjoy a variety. Almonds are high in calcium, vitamin E, magnesium, potassium, and fiber. Walnuts are the best source of omega-3 fats, but it's best to eat them raw as heat diminishes their omega-3 content; they're also high in poly-unsaturated fats, antioxidants, protein, and fiber. Pecans are the highest of all nuts in antioxidants, and contain vitamin E, potassium, zinc, and fiber. Filberts (hazelnuts) are high in potassium, monounsaturated fats, vitamin E, and antioxidants. Peanuts are high in protein and are a good source of folate. Nuts to you!
- Unsalted nuts are usually found in the baking aisle, while salted nuts are found with the snack foods. Nuts help satisfy hunger, so eat a small serving of nuts (about a handful) 5 times a week.
- Store nuts in a sealed container in the refrigerator, or freeze them. They'll keep for up to a year if stored properly.

Pomegranate Chicken

According to ancient lore, the amount of seeds in the pomegranate is exactly the same number (613) as the mitzvot (good deeds) found in the Torah (the Jewish Bible). If you're curious, count away! This fragrant dish also contains honey, carrots, and apricots—traditional foods served with hope for a sweet and fruitful New Year.

2 medium onions, sliced
2 cups baby carrots (or 2 cups peeled and sliced regular carrots)
2 whole chickens (3-½ lb/1.6 kg each), cut into pieces
1 tsp dried thyme
Kosher salt and freshly ground black pepper
1 cup dried whole apricots, loosely packed
1 cup pitted whole prunes, loosely packed
2 tsp sweet paprika

Marinade:
½ cup pomegranate juice (or juice of 1 pomegranate)
2 cloves garlic (about 2 tsp minced)
Juice and rind of 1 lemon
⅓ cup balsamic vinegar
2 tbsp extra virgin olive oil
2 tbsp honey

1. Spray a large roasting pan with cooking spray. Scatter the onions and carrots in the bottom of the pan. Rinse the chicken well and pat dry with paper towels. Trim the excess fat. Place the chicken on top of the vegetables and sprinkle—under the skin and on top—with thyme, and salt and pepper to taste. Tuck the apricots and prunes between the chicken pieces.

2. Whisk the ingredients for the marinade together in a bowl. (If using the juice of a whole pomegranate, reserve some of the seeds for garnish.) Pour over the chicken and sprinkle with paprika. Cover and marinate in the refrigerator for at least 1 hour or for as long as 2 days.

3. When the chicken is marinated, preheat the oven to 350°F. Cook the chicken, covered, for 1-½ hours or until tender. Uncover and cook for 30 minutes longer, basting occasionally, or until the skin is golden. Remove from the pan from the oven and let cool before refrigerating overnight.

4. About 30 minutes before serving, remove and discard any congealed fat from the chicken. Reheat, covered, for 25 to 30 minutes at 350°F. Transfer the heated chicken to a large serving platter and sprinkle with pomegranate seeds. Serve immediately.

Yield: 12 servings. Keeps for up to 3 days in the refrigerator; reheats well. Freezes well for up to 4 months.

315 calories per serving (without skin), 25.9 g carbohydrate, 2.8 g fiber, 31 g protein, 10 g fat (2.4 g saturated), 90 mg cholesterol, 103 mg sodium, 526 mg potassium, 2 mg iron, 43 mg calcium

Chef's Secrets
- *No Pomegranates?* Substitute either bottled pomegranate or cranberry juice. If desired, sprinkle with toasted pumpkin or sesame seeds at serving time.

Quick Chicken Cacciatore

Dinner's done in 30 minutes! This is perfect when you're short on time and need something wonderful for dinner. It is elegant enough for guests or makes a perfect family meal. Serve it over noodles or rice, or for carb-watchers, spoon it over golden strands of spaghetti squash.

6 boneless, skinless single chicken breasts, cut into thin strips
Salt and freshly ground black pepper
2 tbsp olive oil
3 cloves garlic (1 tbsp minced)
2 medium onions, sliced
1 green pepper, seeded and sliced
1 red pepper, seeded and sliced

3 cups sliced mushrooms

3 cups tomato basil sauce

½ cup red wine

1 tsp dried basil

½ tsp dried oregano

¼ tsp red pepper flakes (optional)

2 tbsp minced fresh basil and/or parsley

1. Rinse the chicken strips and pat dry. Trim the excess fat. Sprinkle chicken with salt and pepper.

2. Heat 1 tbsp oil in a large, deep nonstick skillet or Dutch oven on medium-high heat. Add the chicken strips and garlic; stir-fry until the chicken is no longer pink, about 3 to 4 minutes. Transfer to a bowl.

3. Heat the remaining oil in the pan. Add the onions, peppers, and mushrooms; stir-fry for 4 to 5 minutes or until golden.

4. Return the chicken to the pan. Add the tomato sauce, wine, basil, oregano, and red pepper flakes, if using; mix well. Bring to a simmer, then reduce heat and cover partially. Simmer for 20 minutes or until tender, stirring occasionally. Season with additional salt and pepper. Sprinkle with fresh basil and/or parsley.

Yield: 6 servings. Recipe doubles or triples easily. Keeps for up to 2 days in the refrigerator; reheats well. Freezes well for up to 3 months, but the veggies won't be as crisp when thawed.

317 calories per serving, 19.3 g carbohydrate, 2.1 g fiber, 31 g protein, 10.3 g fat (1.5 g saturated), 73 mg cholesterol, 538 mg sodium, 492 mg potassium, 3 mg iron, 138 mg calcium

Rozie's Freeze with Ease Turkey Chili

(See recipe, page 142)

Saucy Mexican Chicken

Fast and fabulous! My longtime friend Phyllis Levy makes this using fresh pineapple.

6 boneless, skinless chicken breasts, trimmed and cut in 1-inch chunks
2-½ cups chunky salsa (mild, medium, or hot)
14 oz (398 ml) can pineapple tidbits, drained
2 tsp mustard
5–6 drops Tabasco sauce, if desired
2–3 cloves garlic, minced
3 tbsp fresh lemon juice
Sweetener to equal 1 tbsp sugar or honey
12 oz can (341 ml) corn niblets, drained

1. Combine all ingredients except corn in a bowl; mix well. Cover and marinate in the refrigerator for 1 hour. Transfer to a large skillet and heat on medium, until bubbling. Reduce heat and simmer uncovered for 25 minutes, stirring occasionally, until sauce has reduced and is thickened. Add corn and cook 5 minutes longer, until piping hot. Serve over rice.

Yield: 6 servings. Reheats and/or freezes well.

241 calories per serving, 3.5 g fat (0.9 g saturated), 73 mg cholesterol, 30 g protein, 22 g carbohydrate, 553 mg sodium, 477 mg potassium, 2 mg iron, 4 g fiber, 78 mg calcium

Variations

- You can use 1 cup of apricot jam instead of pineapple tidbits, but omit sweetener.
- **Pasta Fasta Fiesta:** Omit pineapple. Simmer a 19 ounce (540 ml) can of red kidney or black beans, drained and rinsed, with chicken/salsa mixture. Perfect with penne or fettuccine.

257

Sesame Chicken Mandarin

Mexican and Oriental flavors blend perfectly in this high fiber, low-fat dish. Nutrition with ease!

  10 oz can (284 ml) mandarin oranges
  2 cups chunky salsa (mild or medium)
  ½ cup orange or 3-fruit marmalade
  1 tsp Dijon mustard
  1 tbsp teriyaki sauce
  2 tbsp rice vinegar or lemon juice
  2–3 cloves garlic, crushed
  6 boneless, skinless chicken breasts, trimmed and cut in 1-inch chunks
  2 cups mushrooms, sliced
  1 cup snow peas, trimmed and cut in 1-inch slices
  3 tbsp toasted sesame seeds

1. Drain oranges, reserving ¼ cup juice. In a large skillet, combine juice with all ingredients except snow peas and sesame seeds. Marinate for 30 minutes. Bring to a boil, reduce heat and simmer uncovered on medium for 25 minutes, stirring occasionally. Add drained mandarins and snow peas. Cook 5 minutes longer, until piping hot. Yummy over rice or noodles. Sprinkle with sesame seeds.

Yield: 6 servings. Reheats and/or freezes well.

290 calories per serving, 3.4 g fat (0.9 g saturated), 73 mg cholesterol, 29 g protein, 30 g carbohydrate, 442 mg sodium, 526 mg potassium, 9 mg iron, 3 g fiber, 82 mg calcium

Variation

- **Sesame Apricot Chicken:** Instead of mandarins, use 1 cup canned apricots, drained and sliced.

Slow Cooker Garlicky Chicken Stew

Your kitchen will smell absolutely wonderful when you make this scrumptious dish! The garlic becomes mild and mellow from the long, slow cooking. You can use less (or more) garlic if you wish and add whatever vegetables you have on hand. This is perfect for a chilly winter day. No slow cooker? Make it in the oven as directed below.

> 1 whole chicken (4 lb/1.8 kg), cut into pieces
> 2 medium onions, sliced
> 8 cloves garlic (don't chop)
> 2 stalks celery, cut into chunks
> 1 green pepper, seeded and cut into chunks
> 2 cups sliced mushrooms
> 2 cups baby carrots (or 4 medium carrots, peeled and cut into chunks)
> 4 medium potatoes, peeled and cut into chunks
> 4 medium sweet potatoes, peeled and cut into chunks
> 1 tsp each dried basil, oregano, and thyme
> ½ tsp cayenne pepper
> Salt and freshly ground black pepper
> ¾ cup ketchup or barbecue sauce
> ¾ cup water
> 2 tbsp lemon juice (preferably fresh)

1. Rinse the chicken well and pat dry with paper towels. Trim the excess fat and remove the skin, if desired.
2. Place the chicken into the slow cooker. Add the onions, garlic, celery, bell pepper, mushrooms, carrots, potatoes, and sweet potatoes. Sprinkle with basil, oregano, thyme, cayenne pepper, and salt and pepper to taste. In a small bowl, combine the ketchup, water, and lemon juice. Pour the mixture over the chicken and vegetables; mix well.
3. Cover and cook on the high setting for 4 to 6 hours, or on the low setting for 8 to 10 hours, until the chicken and vegetables are tender.

Yield: 8 servings. Keeps for up to 3 days in the refrigerator; reheats well. Chicken and vegetables can be frozen for up to 3 months, but don't freeze the potatoes or sweet potatoes or they will become mushy when thawed.

298 calories per serving (without skin), 32.2 g carbohydrate, 6 g fiber, 28 g protein, 6.3 g fat (1.7 g saturated), 73 mg cholesterol, 363 mg sodium, 912 mg potassium, 3 mg iron, 79 mg calcium

Oven Method
- Combine all the ingredients in a large roasting pan sprayed with cooking spray. Cover and bake in a preheated 350°F oven for 1-½ to 2 hours. If desired, uncover and baste occasionally for the last half hour of baking.

Stir-Fry Chicken with Mango and Vegetables

Don't go stir-crazy when you read the list of ingredients for this simple stir-fry. Have everything prepared in advance and ready to cook as this comes together very quickly. Experiment with the variations suggested and enjoy a different dinner every time. Serve with brown rice.

Marinade and Chicken:
1 tbsp soy sauce (low-sodium or regular)
2 tbsp hoisin sauce
1 tsp rice vinegar or lemon juice (preferably fresh)
1 to 2 tsp honey or maple syrup (to taste)
1 clove garlic (about 1 tsp minced)
1 tsp Asian (toasted) sesame oil
⅛ tsp cayenne pepper or red pepper flakes
4 boneless, skinless single chicken breasts, cut into thin strips

Vegetable Mixture:
1 red pepper, cut into thin strips
1 green pepper, seeded and cut into thin strips
1 medium onion, halved and thinly sliced
2 baby bok choy (about 2 cups thinly sliced)

¼ lb (125 g) snow peas, ends trimmed (about 1-½ cups)

2 cloves garlic (about 2 tsp minced)

1 mango, peeled and cut into chunks (or 1 cup frozen mango chunks)

1 tbsp canola or peanut oil

1 tbsp cornstarch dissolved in ¼ cup orange juice (preferably fresh)
   or mango juice

1. For the marinade, combine the soy sauce, hoisin sauce, vinegar, honey, garlic, sesame oil, and cayenne pepper in a large bowl. Rinse the chicken breasts and pat dry. Trim the excess fat. Add the chicken breasts to the marinade and mix well. (Can be prepared in advance and marinated up to 2 days in the refrigerator, stirring occasionally.)

2. Prepare the peppers, onion, bok choy, snow peas, and garlic; place on a large platter. Place mango on a separate plate. (If desired, prepare in advance up to this point and refrigerate overnight.)

3. Heat the oil in a nonstick wok or large skillet over high heat. Drain the chicken, reserving the marinade, and stir-fry for 2 minutes, or until chicken is white. Add the vegetables and stir-fry for 2 minutes longer. Stir in the mango and reserved marinade and bring to a boil. Stir in the cornstarch mixture and cook for 1 to 2 minutes longer or until the sauce is bubbly and thickened. This is best served immediately.

Yield: 4 to 6 servings. Can be reheated in the microwave or in a wok, but vegetables won't be as crunchy. If frozen, vegetables will become soggy when thawed.

296 calories per serving, 26.2 g carbohydrate, 2.9 g fiber, 30 g protein, 8.2 g fat (1.3 g saturated), 73 mg cholesterol, 338 mg sodium, 599 mg potassium, 2 mg iron, 70 mg calcium

Variations

- *Go Nuts:* Stir-fry 1 can (8 oz/250 ml) sliced water chestnuts, rinsed and drained, along with vegetables. Garnish with ¼ cup toasted chopped walnuts, sliced almonds, or sesame seeds.

- *Beef Variation:* Substitute 1-½ lb (750 g) lean boneless beef, cut into strips, for the chicken.
- *Vegetarian Variation:* Substitute 1 lb (500 g) extra-firm tofu, cut into strips, for the chicken.
- **As You Like It Stir-Fry.** Instead of bok choy, substitute thinly sliced cabbage. Instead of bell peppers, substitute 2 cups sliced mushrooms. Instead of snow peas, use pea pods or green peas. Instead of mango, substitute 1 cup pineapple tidbits or mandarin orange segments.

Sweet and Sour Stuffed Peppers

Sheila Denton suggested adding honey and lemon juice to the sauce. A grated apple can be added.

> 6 peppers (green and/or red)
> 1-½ lb (750 g) lean ground turkey breast
> 2 egg whites (or 1 egg)
> 1 onion, minced
> ½ tsp salt
> ¼ tsp pepper
> ½ tsp dried basil
> ½ cup uncooked rice
> 2 cups tomato sauce
> ¼ cup honey
> ¼ cup lemon juice
> 1 bay leaf

1. Cut tops off the peppers; carefully remove seeds and cores. Bring a large pot of water to a boil. Add peppers and simmer for 5 minutes, until softened. Drain well. Meanwhile, combine ground turkey with egg whites, onion, seasonings, and rice.

2.   Combine tomato sauce, honey, lemon juice, and bay leaf in a large pot; bring to a boil. Add ½ cup of sauce to the turkey mixture. Stuff the peppers and place them in a single layer in the pot. Reduce heat and simmer covered for 1-½ to 2 hours, basting occasionally. Discard bay leaf.

Yield: 6 servings. These reheat and/or freeze well.

291 calories per serving, 1.2 g fat (0.3 g saturated), 70 mg cholesterol, 32 g protein, 38 g carbohydrate, 784 mg sodium, 838 mg potassium, 3 mg iron, 3 g fiber, 44 mg calcium

Tipsy Apricot Chicken

You'll flip over this sweet and juicy chicken—it's tip-top! This scrumptious dish was a favorite of my friend, the late Bev Gordon, of Richmond Hill. In the winter, make it with dried apricots or canned peaches, and in the summer, use fresh nectarines or peaches.

1 whole chicken (3-½ lb/1.6 kg), cut into pieces
1 cup baby carrots (or 2 medium carrots, peeled and cut into chunks)
1 cup dried whole apricots (or canned sliced peaches, rinsed and drained)
Salt, freshly ground black pepper, and paprika

Sauce:
¼ cup peach schnapps or orange liqueur
¼ cup orange marmalade (low-sugar or all-fruit)
½ cup orange juice (preferably fresh)
1 tbsp hoisin sauce

1.   Preheat the oven to 350°F. Spray a 9- by 13-inch glass baking dish with cooking spray.
2.   Rinse the chicken pieces and pat dry with paper towels. Trim the excess fat. Place the carrots and apricots in the bottom of the baking dish. Arrange the chicken pieces on top. Season the chicken on all sides with salt, pepper, and paprika to taste.

263

3. In a medium saucepan over high heat, combine the schnapps, marmalade, orange juice, and hoisin sauce; stir to mix well and bring to a boil. Pour the hot sauce evenly over the chicken, carrots, and apricots.

4. Roast, uncovered, basting frequently, for about 1 to 1-¼ hours or until the chicken is glazed and golden.

Yield: 6 servings. Keeps for up to 3 days in the refrigerator; reheats well. Freezes well for up to 4 months.

316 calories per serving (without skin), 26.2 g carbohydrate, 2.1 g fiber, 30 g protein, 7.8 g fat (2.1 g saturated), 90 mg cholesterol, 143 mg sodium, 524 mg potassium, 2 mg iron, 34 mg calcium

Tuscan Grilled Chicken Salad
(See recipe, page 143)

■ BEEF AND VEAL

Beef is generally fattier than poultry or fish, so use small amounts along with lots of vegetables. legumes, and grains to achieve a high fiber diet.

Beef, Bean and Barley Cholent

Cholent, a traditional Jewish dish served on the Sabbath, is a slow-cooked casserole that gets its name from the French "chaud" (hot) and "lent" (slow). Because observant Jews are forbidden from turning on an oven or lighting a fire on the Sabbath (from sunset on Friday until sunset on Saturday), cholent must be almost completely cooked before Shabbat begins. This highly nutritious meal-in-a-pot is true comfort food.

> 1 cup mixed dried beans such as kidney beans, white navy beans, or chickpeas
> 3 cups cold water (for soaking)
> 2 tbsp olive or canola oil

3 medium onions, chopped

2 stalks celery, chopped

4 to 6 cloves garlic, coarsely chopped

2 lb (1 kg) lean stewing beef, cut into 1-inch cubes

1 cup pearl barley, rinsed and drained

1 tbsp sweet or Hungarian paprika

2 large sweet potatoes, peeled and cut into chunks (about 4 cups)

4 medium carrots, peeled and cut into chunks (or 2 cups baby carrots)

½ cup ketchup

8 cups water (approximately)

1 tbsp sea salt or Kosher salt (or to taste)

½ tsp freshly ground black pepper

1. Place the beans in a colander and rinse well under cold running water. Transfer to a bowl and add 3 cups water. Soak for 8 hours or preferably overnight. When fully soaked, drain the beans and rinse well.

2. Preheat the oven to 250°F. Heat the oil on medium high heat in a large pot or Dutch oven. Add the onions, celery, and garlic, and brown for 5 minutes. Toss in the stewing beef and cook for 5 minutes longer, stirring often, until the meat is no longer pink.

3. Add the drained beans, barley, paprika, sweet potatoes, carrots, and ketchup to the pot. Pour in enough water to cover the beef-and-vegetable mixture completely (the water should nearly reach the top of the pot). Season with salt and pepper and bring to a boil. Cover the pot tightly and immediately transfer to the oven. Cook overnight and serve for Shabbat lunch.

Yield: 10 servings. Although leftovers can be refrigerated for a day or two, it's best to transform them into soup. (See Chef's Secrets page 266.)

353 calories per serving, 42.7 g carbohydrate, 8.7 g fiber, 25 g protein, 9.7 g fat (2.8 g saturated), 56 mg cholesterol, 691 mg sodium, 773 mg potassium, 10 mg iron, 65 mg calcium

Slow Cooker Cholent

- Soak and drain the beans as directed in Step 1. Reduce the oil to 1 tbsp. Place all the ingredients in a slow cooker that has been sprayed with cooking spray, adding the ingredients in the order listed. Water should come almost to the top of the slow cooker. Cover and cook on the high setting for 6 hours. Before Shabbat, turn the heat setting to low and cook overnight or until ready to serve. Slow cooker disposable liners help save on clean-up and there's no need to spray with cooking spray.

Variation

- Add 1 or 2 parsnips or turnips, cut in chunks. Omit the ketchup and add dried thyme and/or basil, 1 can (28 oz/796 ml) tomatoes, and ½ to 1 cup dry red wine. Pour in enough water (approximately 4 cups) to nearly reach the top of the pot.

Chef's Secrets

- *Leftovers?* Transform leftover cholent into soup! Just combine with an equal amount of water or broth and simmer for 10 minutes. A soup-er idea!
- *Salt Alert!* If sodium is a concern, use low-sodium ketchup and replace salt with a salt substitute.

Italian Style Veal Stew

Easy and tasty. Enjoy!

1 large onion, chopped
3–4 tbsp water
2 cloves garlic, minced
2 stalks celery, chopped
1 green pepper, chopped
1 red pepper, chopped
1–2 tbsp olive oil
2 lb (1 kg) lean veal stewing meat, in 1-inch cubes

1 cup dry white wine

3 tbsp tomato paste

1 tsp salt

Freshly ground pepper

½ tsp dried basil

½ tsp dried oregano

4 carrots, scraped, trimmed, and cut in chunks

5–6 potatoes, peeled and cut into chunks

1. Spray the bottom of a large heavy-bottomed pot with nonstick spray. Heat pan briefly on medium heat. Add onions and water. Cook onions on medium heat for 5 minutes, adding water if necessary to prevent sticking. Stir in garlic, celery, and peppers; cook 5 minutes longer. Remove from pot.

2. Add oil to pot and heat briefly. Add meat and sear quickly on all sides. Add cooked veggies back to pan. Stir in wine, tomato paste, and seasonings; cover and simmer for 45 minutes. Stir occasionally. Add carrots and potatoes; simmer ½ hour longer, until tender. Season to taste.

Yield: 6 servings. Leftovers taste terrific the next day. If freezing, omit potatoes.

388 calories per serving, 11.1 g fat (3.7 g saturated), 123 mg cholesterol, 32 g protein, 34 g carbohydrate, 579 mg sodium, 993 mg potassium, 2 mg iron, 5 g fiber, 74 mg calcium

Variations

- *No wine? No problem!* Use chicken or vegetable broth plus 2 tbsp lemon juice to make 1 cup.
- *Leftover Tomato Paste?* Combine with an equal amount of water and use instead of tomato sauce in another recipe! Or drop tomato paste by tablespoons onto a pan lined with wax paper, cover, and freeze. Add frozen blobs of tomato paste to recipes that call for a couple of tablespoons.
- *Variation:* Omit potatoes. Add 3 zucchini, cut up, during the last 20 minutes of cooking. Serve over fettuccine, penne, or rice.

- *Vegetarian Version:* Omit veal. Add extra vegetables (e.g., mushrooms, squash, turnip, sweet potato, and/or zucchini chunks) along with carrots and potatoes. If desired, add canned beans or chickpeas, well rinsed and drained, during the last 10 minutes of cooking.
- Seitan (a meat analog made from wheat) can be used instead of veal. Cut it into 1-inch chunks and increase cooking time to 1-½ hours. Prepared seitan is available in some natural food shops.
- **Beef Bourguignon:** Substitute lean stewing beef for veal. In Step 1, use 2 cups sliced mushrooms instead of peppers. In Step 2, use red wine instead of white (or use ½ cup red wine and ½ cup beef broth). Instead of basil and oregano, add 1 tsp dried thyme and 1 bay leaf. Simmer covered for 2 hours. Add carrots and potatoes and simmer ½ hour longer. One serving contains 403 calories, 13 g fat (4.3 g saturated) and 94 mg cholesterol.

Secret Ingredient Sweet and Sour Meatballs

Ground chickpeas are the secret ingredient, and no one will know unless you tell! Chickpeas, carrots, and oatmeal add soluble fiber. They also lower the fat content and cost. You can double the meat mixture without doubling the sauce.

1 lb (500 g) extra-lean ground beef, veal, minced turkey, or chicken
1 cup canned chickpeas, drained and rinsed
2 cloves garlic
1 medium onion
1 large carrot
2 egg whites (or 1 whole egg)
½ tsp salt, optional
¼ tsp pepper
½ tsp dried basil
⅔ cup quick-cooking oats or bread crumbs
2 tbsp ketchup, if desired

Sweet and Sour Sauce:
3 cups vegetarian spaghetti sauce (store-bought or homemade)
1 cup water
⅓ cup brown sugar, packed (to taste)
2 tbsp lemon juice or vinegar
Pepper and basil, to taste

1. Place meat in a large mixing bowl. Process chickpeas, garlic, onion, and carrot in the processor until fine, about 20 seconds. Blend in egg whites. Add to meat along with remaining ingredients for meat mixture. Mix lightly to blend. Shape into 1-inch balls, wetting your hands for easier handling. You will have about 60 balls.

2. Bake meatballs uncovered in a single layer on a lightly greased baking sheet at 350°F for 20 minutes (or microwave on HIGH for 5 to 7 minutes, shaking pan to mix meatballs at half time). Meatballs should be lightly cooked and fat will have drained out of the meat.

3. Combine sauce, water, brown sugar, lemon juice, and spices in a large pot. Heat until simmering. Add drained meatballs, cover partially and simmer for 45 minutes, stirring occasionally.

Yield: Serves 10 as a main dish or 15 to 20 as hors d'oeuvres. Reheats and/or freezes well.

218 calories per serving, 7.6 g fat (2.1 g saturated), 17 mg cholesterol, 14 g protein, 25 g carbohydrate, 619 mg sodium, 575 mg potassium, 3 mg iron, 4 g fiber, 48 mg calcium

Chef's Secrets

- *Fat Saving Secrets!* Nutrients are calculated using extra-lean ground beef. Veal contains similar calories and fat. Ground chicken and turkey usually contain fat. Your leanest choice is skinless turkey or chicken breast. Grind it yourself, or have the butcher do it. One serving of turkey meatballs (about 6 meatballs) contains 195 calories and 4 g fat (0.6 g saturated).
- Serve meatballs with pasta, rice, or bulgur. Peas and carrots add color and fiber.

Variations

- **Secret Ingredient Hamburgers:** Prepare meat mixture as directed in Step 1. Shape into 8 patties. Broil or grill burgers for 6 to 8 minutes per side, depending on thickness, until fully cooked.
- **New-Fashioned Cabbage Rolls in Cranberry Sauce:** Lean minced chicken or turkey replaces fatty ground beef and cranberry sauce adds fabulous flavor to the sauce. You can also add a grated apple and a handful of raisins to the sauce.

■ PASTA

Whole-wheat pasta makes all pasta high in fiber.

Broccoli Pasta Quickie

(See recipe, page 145)

Cheater's Hi-Fiber Pasta Sauce

Great when you're in a hurry. Just combine a can of lentils, a jar of sauce, and a splash of wine. Yum!

> 1 cup cooked lentils (or canned, rinsed and well-drained)
> 1 jar vegetarian spaghetti sauce (about 3 cups)
> ¼ cup water
> 1–2 tbsp red or white wine, if desired

1. Process lentils in your food processor until puréed. Add spaghetti sauce and process until well-mixed, scraping down sides of bowl as needed. Combine puréed mixture with water and wine (if using) in a large saucepan. Bring to a boil and simmer partially covered for 10 minutes (or microwave uncovered on HIGH for 10 minutes), stirring occasionally.

Yield: About 4 cups sauce. Freezes and/or reheats well.

101 calories per ½ cup serving, 3.7 g fat (0.5 g saturated), 0 mg cholesterol, 4 g protein, 15 g carbohydrate, 499 mg sodium, 521 mg potassium, 2 mg iron, 4 g fiber, 29 mg calcium

Chef's Secrets
- If using this sauce in dishes that require further cooking, don't bother precooking the sauce.
- To use sauce over spaghetti, simmer the sauce while pasta is cooking. If desired, stir some frozen mixed vegetables into the sauce for extra nutrients. They'll defrost and cook with the sauce!
- If you have time, sauté some onions, peppers, mushrooms, and/or zucchini in a little olive oil or vegetable broth. Combine veggies with sauce ingredients and simmer uncovered for 10 minutes.

Fasta Pasta
(See recipe, page 145)

Hi-Fiber Vegetarian Lasagna
(See recipe, page 146)

High-Fiber Vegetarian Pasta Sauce
Adding mashed kidney beans or lentils to the sauce will thicken it, as well as increase the fiber content. No one will know! This is an excellent sauce to serve over spiral pasta such as fusilli or rotini. I also love to use it as a sauce for chicken breasts or tofu.

1 tbsp olive or vegetable oil
1 large onion, chopped
1 green pepper, chopped
1 red pepper, chopped
4 cloves garlic, crushed
3 medium zucchini, chopped (1 lb/500 g)

2 cups mushrooms, sliced
4 large fresh tomatoes, roughly chopped
2 cans (5½ oz/156 ml) tomato paste
2-⅔ cups water
Salt, to taste
½ tsp pepper
1 tsp dried basil
1 tsp sugar
19 oz (540 ml) can red kidney beans or lentils, rinsed, drained, and mashed

1. *Conventional Method:* Heat oil in a large, heavy-bottomed pot. Sauté onion and peppers for 5 minutes on medium heat. Add garlic, zucchini, and mushrooms and sauté 5 minutes longer. Add tomatoes and cook 3 minutes more. Add remaining ingredients and mix well. Bring to a boil. Simmer partly covered for 20 to 25 minutes, stirring occasionally.
2. *Microwave Method:* Combine oil, onions and peppers in a 3-quart microsafe casserole. Microwave covered on HIGH for 3 minutes. Add garlic, zucchini, and mushrooms. Microwave 3 minutes more. Add tomatoes and microwave 3 minutes. Stir in remaining ingredients. Cover and microwave on HIGH for 20 minutes, stirring once or twice.

Yield: About 8 cups (8 servings). Freezes well.

171 calories per serving, 2.7 g fat (0.3 g saturated), 0 mg cholesterol, 8 g protein, 32 g carbohydrate, 44 mg sodium, 777 mg potassium, 2 mg iron, 10 g fiber, 38 mg calcium

Chef's Secrets
- If you substitute 28 oz (796 ml) canned tomatoes for fresh tomatoes, decrease water to 1-⅓ cups.
- If you have trouble digesting legumes, omit them. Instead, thicken sauce with oats, a super source of soluble fiber. Stir ⅓ cup of quick-cooking oats into sauce during the last 5 minutes of cooking.
- If desired, purée all or part of the cooked sauce in batches in the food processor.

Many Color Vegetable Lasagna

There are several steps to this excellent recipe, but it's really quite easy to make. It's a favorite of my catering clients. So many vegetables, so many vitamins! Packed with potassium, calcium, and fiber.

4 cups tomato sauce (homemade or bottled)

So-Low Alfredo Sauce (page 286)

9 lasagna noodles, cooked, drained, and laid flat on towels

2 onions, sliced

3 or 4 cloves garlic, crushed

2 green and 2 red peppers, cut into strips

2 zucchini, sliced on an angle ½-inch thick

2 cups mushrooms, sliced

3 cup frozen California mixed vegetables (or 1 cup each of fresh broccoli, cauliflower, and carrots, cut up)

2 cups grated low-fat mozzarella cheese

1. Cook sauces as directed. (They can be prepared in advance and refrigerated for up to 2 days.) Prepare lasagna noodles.

2. In a large microwave casserole or glass bowl, combine onions, garlic, and peppers. Cover and microwave on HIGH for 5 minutes, until tender-crisp. Add zucchini and mushrooms and microwave covered on HIGH 3 to 4 minutes longer. (Alternately, sauté onions, garlic, and peppers in a little oil in a nonstick skillet until golden. Add zucchini and mushrooms and cook 5 minutes longer.)

3. In another microwave casserole or glass bowl, microwave frozen mixed vegetables covered on HIGH for 5 to 7 minutes, until tender-crisp. (If using fresh vegetables, sprinkle them with a little water before microwaving. Alternately, cook veggies in a saucepan for 8 minutes.) Combine all the vegetables and mix gently.

4. Place ⅓ of the tomato sauce in the bottom of a lightly greased or sprayed 9- by 13-inch casserole. Arrange 3 lasagna noodles in a single layer over

273

sauce. Top with half of the Alfredo Sauce. Arrange half the vegetables over the sauce. Sprinkle lightly with ⅔ cup of cheese. Repeat once more. Top with remaining noodles and tomato sauce. Sprinkle with cheese. (Can be made in advance up to this point and refrigerated.)

5. Bake uncovered in a preheated 375°F oven for 40 to 45 minutes. Let stand for 10 to 15 minutes for easier cutting.

Yield: 12 servings. Freezes and/or reheats well.

275 calories per serving, 7.3 g fat (4 g saturated), 21 mg cholesterol, 16 g protein, 39 g carbohydrate, 268 mg sodium, 727 mg potassium, 3 mg iron, 6 g fiber, 339 mg calcium

Mexican Pasta with Beans
(See recipe, page 147)

Pasta Primavera
(See recipe, page 148)

Pasta Primavera Lite-Style
The microwave makes this family favorite quick and easy to prepare. It's delicious hot or cold!

12 oz pkg (340 g) spiral pasta
1 onion, cut into 1-inch chunks
1 green and 1 red pepper, cut into 1-inch chunks
2 cups broccoli florets
1 cup sliced carrots
3–4 cloves garlic, minced
1 cup snow peas, tails removed
1 cup sliced zucchini
Skinny Parmesan Sauce (page 285)

1. Cook pasta according to package directions. Drain and rinse well. Combine veggies in a covered microsafe casserole. Sprinkle with 2 tbsp water. Microwave covered on HIGH for 6 to 7 minutes, until tender-crisp, stirring at half time.
2. Prepare sauce. Mix together with pasta and vegetables. Place in a sprayed 3-quart casserole. If desired, thin with a little skim milk. (Can be made ahead and refrigerated.) Cover with waxed or parchment paper. Microwave on HIGH for 5 minutes (10 minutes if refrigerated), until piping hot. (Alternately, bake uncovered at 350°F for 25 minutes.) Adjust seasonings to taste.

Yield: 6 to 8 servings. Freezes well. Delicious cold as a pasta salad! Just thin with a little skim milk.

326 calories per serving, 6 g fat (3.1 g saturated), 18 mg cholesterol, 15 g protein, 53 g carbohydrate, 246 mg sodium, 466 mg potassium, 3 mg iron, 5 g fiber, 262 mg calcium

Variations
- **Tortellini Primavera:** Substitute cheese or spinach tortellini for spiral pasta.
- *Time-Saving Secret!* Substitute 4 cups of frozen California mixed vegetables for fresh vegetables.

Penne Al Pesto Jardinière

The starchy cooking liquid binds with the cheese to thicken the sauce. So pretty with 3-color pasta!

1 lb penne (ziti, fusilli, or rotini can be used)
1 onion, halved and cut in strips
4 peppers, (green, red, yellow and/or orange), halved, seeded, and cut in strips
2 zucchini, cut in strips
3 cloves garlic, crushed
1-½ tbsp olive oil

3–4 tbsp balsamic vinegar or lemon juice
Salt and pepper, to taste
¼ cup grated Parmesan cheese
½ cup fresh basil, finely chopped
1-½–2 cups tomato sauce (bottled or homemade)
1 chopped tomato, to garnish
Parmesan cheese, to garnish

1. Preheat oven to 425°F. Prepare vegetables and place on a sprayed (or nonstick) baking sheet. Add garlic, olive oil, and vinegar. Sprinkle lightly with salt and pepper and mix well. Roast vegetables uncovered at 425°F for 20 minutes, until nicely browned.
2. Meanwhile, bring a large pot of salted water to a boil. Cook pasta according to package directions, about 10 minutes, until al dente. Ladle out a little of the cooking liquid just before draining pasta. Drain pasta but do not rinse.
3. Return pasta to saucepan. Add Parmesan, basil, and about ¼ cup of reserved cooking liquid; mix well. Add tomato sauce and roasted vegetables. Adjust seasonings to taste. Cook briefly, just until heated through. Garnish with diced tomato and sprinkle with a light dusting of Parmesan cheese, if desired. Great hot or at room temperature.

Yield: 8 main dish servings. Reheats well. If frozen, vegetables may lose some of their texture.

267 calories per serving, 4.6 g fat (1.1 g saturated), 3 mg cholesterol, 9 g protein, 48 g carbohydrate, 342 mg sodium, 434 mg potassium, 3 mg iron, 4 g fiber, 77 mg calcium

Variation

- **Penne with Roasted Vegetable Purée:** In Step 2, reserve about a cup of the cooking liquid from pasta. In Step 3, process 2 cups of the roasted vegetables until smooth. Add ½ cup of reserved cooking liquid to thin the mixture; process briefly. (If necessary, add a little more liquid.) Stir purée into pasta along with remaining ingredients. (This is a great way to get kids to eat their veggies!)

276

Penne Pesto with Tuna and Veggies
(See recipe, page 150)

Penne with Roasted Peppers and Sun-Dried Tomatoes
(See recipe, page 152)

Pesto Pasta Salad
(See recipe, page 153)

Rotini with Dried Mushrooms and Chunky Vegetables

5 quarts water

½ cup dried mushrooms plus 1 cup water for soaking

1 lb (500 g) rotini (spirals)

1 tbsp olive oil

2 onions, cut into chunks

1 red pepper, cut into strips

1 yellow or green pepper, cut into strips

2–3 cloves garlic, sliced

3–4 tbsp dry white wine

28 oz can (796 ml) canned tomatoes

1 tsp dried basil

¼ tsp dried thyme

Salt and pepper, to taste

½ cup grated Parmesan cheese, to garnish

1. Put water for the pasta up to boil. Soak mushrooms in 1 cup of hot water for 20 to 30 minutes. Drain well, reserving the soaking water. Chop mushrooms into ½-inch pieces.
2. Heat oil in a large, nonstick skillet. Add onions and peppers. Sauté for 5

minutes on medium-high heat. Add garlic and mushrooms and cook for 3 or 4 minutes more. Stir in wine and cook until wine evaporates, 2 to 3 minutes more. Add canned tomatoes, soaking water from the mushrooms and seasonings. Break up tomatoes, bring to a boil and reduce heat. Simmer uncovered for 10 to 15 minutes, stirring occasionally.

3.   Meanwhile, cook pasta according to package directions. Drain pasta but do not rinse; reserve a little of the cooking water. Combine cooking water with pasta and sauce; mix well. Adjust seasonings to taste. Sprinkle with grated cheese.

Yield: 6 to 8 servings. Reheats well.

359 calories per serving, 6.3 g fat (2.2 g saturated), 7 mg cholesterol, 14 g protein, 61 g carbohydrate, 368 mg sodium, 457 mg potassium, 4 mg iron, 5 g fiber, 184 mg calcium

Variation

- Put pasta and sauce in a lightly greased casserole. Instead of Parmesan cheese, sprinkle with 1 cup grated low-fat mozzarella cheese. Bake uncovered at 350°F for 20 to 25 minutes, until bubbling and cheese has melted.

■ MARINADES AND SAUCES

Many of the following recipes are needed to complete some of the dishes in this book. But they'll work great in your own creations, too.

Apricot Hoisin Marinade

Oy, this hoisin-based marinade is soy sinful! It's wonderful on chicken, meat, fish, or tofu. A food processor speeds up preparation, so why not make a double batch?

> 1 small slice peeled fresh ginger (about 2 tsp minced)
> 3 cloves garlic
> 3 green onions, cut in 2-inch pieces
> ⅓ cup hoisin sauce
> ⅓ cup apricot jam (low-sugar or all-fruit)
> 2 tbsp soy sauce (low-sodium or regular)
> 2 tbsp rice vinegar or lemon juice (preferably fresh)
> 2 tsp Asian (toasted) sesame oil
> ⅛ tsp red pepper flakes or cayenne
> 1 tsp honey

1. In a food processor fitted with the steel blade, drop the ginger, garlic, and green onions through the feed tube while the motor is running. Process until minced, about 10 seconds.
2. Scrape down the sides of the bowl. Add hoisin sauce, jam, soy sauce, vinegar or lemon juice, sesame oil, pepper flakes, and honey; process for 8 to 10 seconds to blend.
3. Transfer to a container and store, covered, in the refrigerator until ready to use.

Yield: 1-¼ cups. Keeps for up to 1 week in the refrigerator. Freezes well for up to 3 months.

23 calories per tbsp, 4.1 g carbohydrate, 0.2 g fiber, 0 g protein, 0.6 g fat (0.1 g saturated), 0 mg cholesterol, 117 mg sodium, 17 mg potassium, 0 mg iron, 4 mg calcium

Variation
- Instead of apricot jam, substitute orange marmalade or peach jam.

Asian Marinade

This simple marinade is fabulous with fish, chicken, beef, or tofu. Use it to marinate grilled broccoli florets, green beans, asparagus, or portobello mushrooms. This also makes a terrific stir-fry sauce. Soy versatile!

2 cloves garlic
1 small slice peeled fresh ginger (about 2 tsp minced)
2 to 3 tbsp soy sauce (low-sodium or regular)
2 tbsp honey or granular Splenda
2 tbsp orange juice (preferably fresh) or rice vinegar
1 tsp Asian (toasted) sesame oil
½ tsp dried basil
Freshly ground black pepper

1. In a food processor fitted with the steel blade, process the garlic and ginger until minced, about 10 seconds.
2. Scrape down the sides of the bowl. Add the soy sauce, honey, orange juice or vinegar, sesame oil, and basil. Season with pepper to taste. Process until combined, about 5 seconds.
3. Transfer to a container and store, covered, in the refrigerator until ready to use.

Yield: About ½ cup. Recipe can be doubled or tripled. Keeps for up to 1 week in the refrigerator. Freezes well for up to 3 months.

27 calories per tbsp, 5.4 g carbohydrate, 0.1 g fiber, 0 g protein, 0.6 g fat (0.1 g saturated), 0 mg cholesterol, 133 mg sodium, 25 mg potassium, 0 mg iron, 4 mg calcium. If made with Splenda, 1 tbsp contains 18 calories and 2.2 g carbohydrate.

Chef's Secret
- *Ginger Tips:* An easy way to peel fresh ginger is to scrape it with the tip of a spoon.

Teriyaki Marinade

This terrific marinade is guaranteed to bring rave reviews from family and friends. It also does double-duty as a sauce and is delicious on meat, poultry, fish, tofu, or vegetables.

¼ cup orange juice (preferably fresh) or mango juice
¼ cup soy sauce (low-sodium or regular)
2 tbsp lemon juice (preferably fresh)
3 cloves garlic (about 1 tbsp minced)
1 slice peeled fresh ginger (about 1 tbsp minced)
2 tsp Asian (toasted) sesame oil
2 tbsp maple syrup or honey

1. Combine all the ingredients in a jar and shake well. (Or combine in a food processor and process for 8 to 10 seconds until blended.)
2. Store, covered, in the refrigerator, until ready to use.

Yield: About ¾ cup, enough for 2 to 3 lb (1 to 1-½ kg) meat, fish, chicken, or tofu. Keeps for up to 1 week in the refrigerator. Freezes well for up to 3 months.

18 calories per tbsp, 3.1 g carbohydrate, 0.1 g fiber, 0 g protein, 0.7 g fat (0.1 g saturated), 0 mg cholesterol, 146 mg sodium, 28 mg potassium, 0 mg iron, 4 mg calcium

Teriyaki Sauce

Prepare marinade as directed above. Place in a saucepan and heat until boiling. Dissolve 1 tbsp cornstarch in 2 tbsp water or orange juice. Stir the cornstarch solution into the boiling marinade and cook, stirring constantly, until smooth and thickened, about 2 minutes. Serve as a sauce.

Chef's Secrets

- *Timing's Everything!* Marinate meat or poultry for 1 to 2 hours (or up to 48 hours) in the refrigerator. Marinate fish or tofu for 1 hour.

- *Veggie Time!* Marinate vegetables (e.g., asparagus, green beans, or broccoli) for 30 minutes to 2 hours. Drain, reserving the marinade. Grill, steam, or microwave the vegetables. Use the reserved marinade to make Teriyaki Sauce (page 281), and serve it over the grilled or cooked vegetables.

Best-O Pesto

Best-O Pesto is ready "presto" with the help of your processor! My original recipe had 83 calories and over 8 grams of fat per tablespoon. This lighter version has a fraction of the fat!

2 tbsp pine nuts (or walnuts)
2 cups tightly packed fresh basil leaves
½ cup fresh parsley
4 cloves garlic, peeled
2–3 tbsp grated Parmesan cheese
2 tbsp olive oil (extra virgin is best)
¼ cup tomato juice or vegetable broth
Salt and pepper, to taste

1. Place nuts in a small skillet and brown over medium heat for 2 to 3 minutes. Wash basil and parsley; dry thoroughly. Start the processor and drop garlic through feed tube. Process until minced. Add nuts, basil, parsley, and Parmesan cheese. Process until fine, about 15 seconds. Drizzle oil and juice through the feed tube while the machine is running. Process until blended. Season to taste.

Yield: 1 cup. Pesto keeps for 4 or 5 days in the refrigerator, or can be frozen for 2 months.

27 calories per tbsp, 2.4 g fat (0.5 g saturated), <1 mg cholesterol, <1 g protein, <1 g carbohydrate, 30 mg sodium, 52 mg potassium, trace iron, trace fiber, 23 mg calcium

Chef's Secrets

- When basil is expensive, use a combination of fresh basil and fresh spinach. It works perfectly!
- Freeze pesto in ice cube trays. Transfer them to a plastic bag and store in the freezer. Each cube contains 2 tablespoons pesto. Add a cube or two to your favorite pasta sauce, soup, or vegetarian stew.
- A couple of spoonfuls of pesto added to pasta salad or vinaigrette dressing will enhance the flavor.

Peanut Sauce

This Szechuan-inspired sauce is scrumptious on chicken, beef, fish, or tofu. Try it in stir-fries or on steamed veggies such as broccoli, cauliflower, or carrots. You'll go nuts over it!

3 cloves garlic (about 1 tbsp minced)
1 slice peeled fresh ginger (about 1 tbsp minced)
3 tbsp soy sauce (low-sodium or regular)
½ cup natural peanut butter
2 tbsp honey (or to taste)
2 tbsp rice vinegar
2 tsp Asian (toasted) sesame oil
¼ tsp cayenne pepper

1. In a food processor fitted with the steel blade, drop the garlic and ginger through the feed tube while the motor is running; process until minced, about 10 seconds.
2. Add the soy sauce, peanut butter, honey, vinegar, sesame oil, and cayenne; process until blended, about 15 seconds. Scrape down the sides of bowl if needed. If the sauce is too thick, thin with a little water.

Yield: About 1 cup. Keeps for up to 2 months in the refrigerator. Reheat gently but don't boil or the sauce may separate. Don't freeze.

58 calories per tbsp, 3.9 g carbohydrate, 0.5 g fiber, 2 g protein, 4.0 g fat (0.5 g satu-rated), 0 mg cholesterol, 115 mg sodium, 10 mg potassium, 0 mg iron, 2 mg calcium

Quick 'n' Easy Tomato Sauce (Vegetarian Spaghetti Sauce)

This sauce is a quick and easy substitute for the bottled version! To make it fat-free, omit olive oil.

28 oz can (796 ml) tomatoes (stewed, whole, or crushed)

5-½ oz can (156 ml) tomato paste

1 tsp olive oil (preferably extra virgin)

3 cloves garlic, crushed

Salt and pepper, to taste

¼ tsp cayenne or red pepper flakes

½ tsp oregano

1 tbsp fresh basil, minced (or ½ tsp dried)

½ tsp sugar

1–2 tbsp red or white wine, optional

1. Combine all ingredients in a large saucepan or covered microsafe casserole, breaking up tomatoes if necessary. To microwave, cook covered on HIGH for 10 minutes, stirring at half time. To cook conventionally, bring sauce to a boil, reduce heat and simmer covered for 20 to 25 minutes, stirring occasionally. Adjust seasonings to taste.

Yield: Approximately 4 cups sauce. Reheats and/or freezes well. Freeze in 1 cup portions.

43 calories per ½ cup serving, 0.8 g fat (0.1 g saturated), 0 mg cholesterol, 2 g protein, 9 g carbohydrate, 27 mg sodium, 413 mg potassium, 1 mg iron, 2 g fiber, 40 mg calcium

Variations
- If you are sodium-sensitive, use canned tomatoes and tomato paste without added salt.
- **Sun-Dried Tomato Sauce:** Soak ½ cup sun-dried tomatoes (dry pack) in boiling water for 10 minutes, until soft. Drain well; chop coarsely. Add to sauce ingredients and cook as directed.
- **Light 'n' Easy Meat Sauce:** Sauté 1 onion, 1 green pepper and 2 cloves crushed garlic in 2 tbsp water until tender (or microwave on HIGH for 3 minutes). Add 1 lb lean ground turkey and cook until it loses its pink color, stirring occasionally (about 5 to 6 minutes in the microwave). Add remaining ingredients and simmer covered for about 1 hour (or 20 minutes on HIGH in the microwave). Stir occasionally. Adjust seasonings to taste. Makes about 6 cups of sauce. Half a cup of sauce contains about 91 calories and 3.7 g fat (1 g saturated).
- *Fiber Facts:* Add a finely grated carrot to the sauce for fiber and natural sweetness. For additional fiber and a "meaty" texture, add 2 to 3 tbsp of quick-cooking oats to the sauce 5 minutes before the end of cooking. If the cooked sauce is too thick, thin it with a little water or wine.
- Most pasta sauces freeze beautifully. Pack in 1 cup containers for convenience, leaving about ½-inch space at the top to allow for expansion. When you need some sauce, place the frozen container under running water briefly. Pop out the contents and transfer them to a microsafe bowl. Thaw on HIGH power. (DEFROST takes too long!) Stir several times. One cup of sauce takes about 5 minutes to thaw and heat.

Skinny Parmesan Sauce

This is an excellent light sauce to use with pasta, vegetables, or fish.

2 tsp butter, margarine, or oil
3 tbsp flour
1-½ cups skim milk or vegetable broth
1 bay leaf, if desired

½ cup grated Parmesan cheese

2 tbsp minced fresh basil (or 1 tsp dried)

Salt and pepper, to taste

¼ tsp grated nutmeg

1.   Combine butter and flour in a 4-cup glass measuring cup. Microwave on HIGH for 30 seconds. Gradually whisk in milk or broth. Add bay leaf. Microwave on HIGH 4 to 4-½ minutes, until bubbling, whisking twice during cooking. Discard bay leaf. Stir in cheese and seasonings.

Yield: About 2 cups sauce (8 servings of ¼ cup).

71 calories per ¼ cup serving, 3.6 g fat (2.2 g saturated), 13 mg cholesterol, 5 g protein, 5 g carbohydrate, 164 mg sodium, 83 mg potassium, trace iron, trace fiber, 158 mg calcium

Variations

- **Lactose-Free Skinny Sauce:** Prepare Skinny Parmesan Sauce as directed but use non-dairy margarine or oil instead of butter. Use vegetable broth, soy milk, or lactose-free milk as your liquid. Eliminate Parmesan cheese. Add a dash of basil and oregano to sauce.
- **Cheese Sauce:** Prepare Skinny Parmesan Sauce but omit nutmeg and Parmesan cheese. Stir ⅓ cup grated low-fat Cheddar cheese and ½ teaspoon dried mustard into sauce.

So-Low Alfredo Sauce

An excellent source of calcium.

2 tbsp cornstarch

1-¾ cups skim milk

3 cloves garlic, crushed

⅓ cup grated Parmesan cheese

3–4 tbsp light cream cheese

Salt and pepper, to taste
2–3 tbsp minced fresh basil (or 1 tsp dried)
¼ tsp nutmeg

1.   Blend cornstarch with milk until smooth. Add garlic and microwave on
     HIGH for 4 to 5 minutes, until thick, stirring 2 or 3 times. Whisk in
     remaining ingredients until smooth. Makes 2 cups sauce.

*56 calories per ¼ cup serving, 2.5 g fat (1.5 g saturated), 10 mg cholesterol, 4 g
protein, 4 g carbohydrate, 117 mg sodium, 91 mg potassium, trace iron, trace fiber,
125 mg calcium*

Variation

•   **Pesto Alfredo Sauce:** Add 3 tbsp Best-O Pesto (page 282). Great over
    fettuccine.

Tahini Sauce

Although tahini is fairly high in calories, it's necessary for authentic Israeli-style falafel!

½ cup tahini (sesame paste, available in Middle Eastern and health food
   stores)
¾ cup water
1 clove garlic, crushed
½ tbsp fresh lemon juice (or to taste)
Salt, to taste

1.   Place tahini in a jar. Add water and mix well. Add remaining ingredients
     and shake until blended.

Yield: About 1-¼ cups. Keeps about 2 weeks in the refrigerator. Do not freeze.

*36 calories per tbsp, 3.3 g fat (0.5 g saturated), 0 mg cholesterol, 1 g protein, 1 g
carbohydrate, trace sodium, 28 mg potassium, trace iron, <1 g fiber, 9 mg calcium*

Chef's Secrets

- *Fat-Saving Secret!* Instead of stirring tahini before you measure it, pour off the oil that has risen to the top of the jar and discard it.
- **Tahini Yogurt Sauce:** Combine Tahini Sauce with equal amounts of nonfat yogurt.
- **Baked Fish Middle Eastern Style:** Sprinkle halibut steaks (or any thick, firm fish fillets) with salt and pepper. Spread top side of fish with Tahini Sauce (or Tahini Yogurt Sauce). Place on a sprayed foil-lined pan and bake in a preheated 450°F oven for 12 to 15 minutes.

■ VEGETARIAN ENTRÉES

What with the beans and vegetables that make up most vegetarian dishes, you can really pack in the fiber.

Almost Meat Lasagna

You'll have no "beefs" when you serve this delicious, fiber-packed dish. My friend Bev Binder of Winnipeg makes a marvelous meatless lasagna using ground beef substitute—it looks and tastes like it's made with meat. This adapted version is sure to please everyone, vegetarian or not.

9 or 10 lasagna noodles (preferably whole-wheat)
1 to 2 tbsp olive oil
1 medium onion, chopped
1 red pepper, seeded and chopped
1-½ cups chopped mushrooms
2 cloves garlic (about 2 tsp minced)
1 pkg (12 oz/340 g) vegetarian ground beef substitute
3 cups chunky tomato sauce
1 tsp dried basil
½ tsp dried oregano

3 cups light ricotta cheese

1 pkg (10 oz/300 g) frozen chopped spinach, thawed and squeezed dry

1-¼ cups grated low-fat mozzarella cheese

1. Cook the lasagna noodles according to package directions, but undercook them slightly so they are al dente, not too soft. Drain well and lay flat on a clean towel.

2. Meanwhile, heat the oil in a large, deep nonstick skillet on medium-high heat. Add the onion, red pepper, mushrooms, and garlic and sauté for 5 minutes or until golden. Stir in the ground beef substitute, tomato sauce, basil, and oregano. Continue cooking, uncovered, on medium-high heat for 5 minutes or until the mixture is heated through, stirring occasionally. (If desired, the sauce can be prepared in advance, up to this point, and stored in the refrigerator overnight.)

3. In a large mixing bowl and using an electric mixer, or in a food processor fitted with the steel blade, combine the ricotta cheese and spinach; mix or process well.

4. Spray a 9- by 13-inch glass baking dish with cooking spray. Evenly spread about 1-½ cups sauce in the bottom of the baking dish. Place 3 of the cooked lasagna noodles on top of the sauce and spread half the ricotta cheese mixture on top. Repeat with another layer of sauce, noodles, and ricotta. Top with the last 3 cooked lasagna noodles, sauce, and mozzarella. You'll have 3 layers of sauce and noodles, 2 layers of ricotta cheese, and a topping of mozzarella cheese. (If desired, the lasagna can be prepared in advance up to this point, covered, and refrigerated overnight.)

5. Bake, uncovered, in a preheated 375°F oven for 30 to 40 minutes or until bubbly and golden. Let stand for 10 minutes for easier slicing.

Yield: 8 to 10 servings. Keeps for up to 2 to 3 days; reheats well. Freezes well for up to 3 months.

389 calories per serving, 38.1 g carbohydrate, 9.3 g fiber, 30 g protein, 13 g fat (6.6 g saturated), 40 mg cholesterol, 701 mg sodium, 586 mg potassium, 5 mg iron, 468 mg calcium

Chef's Secrets

- *Almost Meat Sauce:* Prepare the sauce as directed in Step 2 and serve it over your favorite pasta.
- *Where's the Beef?* Soy meat crumbles (which are a ground beef substitute) make a great alternative to ground meat. (One soy brand, Yves Veggie Ground Round, is Kosher and dairy-free.) Soy is an excellent source of protein and fiber, is low in fat, and is cholesterol-free. Use soy ground beef substitutes in pasta sauces, stuffed peppers, casseroles, or chili. Do note, however, that some people may experience "gastric distress"—oy, that soy!
- *Soy Good:* Firm silken tofu can be used instead of ricotta cheese. Omit the mozzarella cheese if you want to make a dairy-free lasagna.

Baked Tofu in BBQ Sauce

Whenever I eat this tasty dish or the terrific variation below, I feel so healthy!

1 lb firm tofu (500 g), sliced ½-inch thick
1-½ cups bottled or homemade BBQ sauce
2 large onions, peeled and sliced
2 cups mushrooms, sliced

1. Preheat oven to 400°F. Place sliced tofu between layers of paper towels on a plate. Top with another plate. Weigh it down with cans and let drain for 20 minutes. Pour half of sauce into a sprayed oblong casserole. Add onions and mushrooms; mix well. Arrange sliced tofu over onion mixture. Top with remaining sauce. Bake uncovered at 400°F for 20 minutes. Turn tofu over with a spatula. Baste with sauce and spoon some of the onion mixture on top. Bake 10 minutes longer.

Yield: 6 servings. This reheats well, but freezing is not recommended. I like to serve it with brown basmati rice. Leftover baked tofu is delicious in sandwiches.

180 calories per serving, 7.9 g fat (1.2 g saturated), 0 mg cholesterol, 14 g protein, 17 g carbohydrate, 522 mg sodium, 420 mg potassium, 9 mg iron, 4 g fiber, 177 mg calcium

Variations

- Use tofu processed with calcium sulphate for maximum calcium intake. This can also be made with light 1% fat extra-firm silken tofu. (This is softer than regular firm tofu.)
- **Terrific Baked Tofu:** Follow recipe above, but omit BBQ sauce. Substitute 1-¼ cups tomato sauce and ¼ cup bottled Szechuan Spicy Duck Sauce or Chinese plum sauce. (If using plum sauce, add ¼ tsp red pepper flakes or a few drops of Tabasco sauce.)

Black Bean and Corn Casserole

Picture perfect! Elegant enough for guests. Full of fiber, full of beans!

4 cups cooked or canned black beans
2 cups stewed tomatoes or tomato sauce
3 tbsp maple syrup or brown sugar
2 medium onions, chopped
1 green pepper, chopped
1 red pepper, chopped
¾ cup canned or frozen corn niblets
1 tsp Dijon mustard
½ tsp each cayenne pepper and chili powder
Freshly ground pepper, to taste

1. Spray a 2-quart ovenproof casserole with nonstick spray. Combine all ingredients and mix well. Bake covered at 350°F for 45 minutes, until bubbling hot and flavors are blended. (Or microwave in a covered microsafe casserole on HIGH for 15 to 18 minutes. Stir once or twice during cooking.)

Yield: 6 servings of about 1 cup each. Freezes and/or reheats well. Also delicious cold.

207 calories per cup, 1 g fat (0.2 g saturated), 0 mg cholesterol, 10 g protein, 42 g carbohydrate, 270 mg sodium, 577 mg potassium, 3 mg iron, 10 g fiber, 62 mg calcium

Chef's Secret
- Serve over rice or pasta with Israeli Salad (page 93), or use as a side dish.

Crustless Zucchini Quiche
(See recipe, page 38)

Curried Chunky Eggplant and Chickpeas

My friend Maurice Borts of Ottawa renamed this dish "Seven-Time Winner" because he's served it seven times and each time the guests asked for the recipe. This makes a big batch but leftovers freeze well. If you have vegetarians at your table, they'll devour this dish.

> 2 medium eggplants
> Salt
> 1 tbsp olive oil
> 1 large red onion (about 2 cups chopped)
> 1 can (19 oz/540 ml) chickpeas, drained and rinsed
> 3 to 4 tsp curry powder
> ½ tsp ground cumin
> ½ cup cold water
> 6 tbsp lemon juice (preferably fresh)
> 2 to 3 tbsp honey (or to taste)
> 2 tbsp ketchup
> Salt and freshly ground black pepper

1. Cut eggplant into ½-inch chunks and measure 8 cups. Place the chopped eggplant into a colander and lightly sprinkle with salt. Let stand for 20 to 30 minutes; rinse well and squeeze gently to remove any excess liquid and bitter juices from the eggplant.

2. Steam the eggplant in a vegetable steamer until tender, about 10 to 12 minutes. (Or cover and microwave in a large microwaveable bowl for 10 minutes, stirring at half time.) Don't overcook.

3.   Heat the oil in a large pot on medium high heat. Add the onion and sauté until tender-crisp, about 6 to 8 minutes. Transfer the steamed eggplant along with the drained chickpeas to the pot; mix well. Add the curry powder, cumin, water, lemon juice, honey, and ketchup; stir to combine and bring to a boil. Reduce heat to low and simmer, uncovered, stirring occasionally, for 8 to 10 minutes. Season with salt and pepper to taste and serve.

Yield: About 6 cups (12 servings of ½ cup each as a side dish). Keeps for up to 3 days in the refrigerator; reheats well. Freezes well for up to 2 months.

104 calories per ½ cup serving, 20.8 g carbohydrate, 3.7 g fiber, 3 g protein, 1.8 g fat (0.2 g saturated), 0 mg cholesterol, 272 mg sodium, 199 mg potassium, 1 mg iron, 26 mg calcium

Chef's Secrets

- *What's in Store:* Eggplants come in all shapes, sizes, colors, and varieties. Choose shiny, smooth, firm eggplants with no soft spots. Avoid those with spongy or brown spots.
- *Size Counts:* Large eggplants tend to be bitter and are often full of seeds. Small, slender eggplants have smaller seeds and are usually more tender. Choose small or medium eggplants for grilling or broiling. Larger ones are fine for making an eggplant spread, but remove the seeds after cooking.
- **Sponge-Blob Eggplant:** Eggplant acts like a sponge, soaking up as much oil as you give it. Salting eggplant before cooking draws out the bitter juices and excess moisture, so it needs less oil and you won't turn into a blob! Smaller varieties usually don't need to be salted before cooking.

Easy BBQ Chickpea Casserole
(See recipe, page 155)

Easy Enchiladas
(See recipe, page 156)

Easy Vegetarian Chili
(See recipe, page 157)

Eggplant Roll-Ups
(See recipe, page 158)

Enchilada Lasagna
(See recipe, page 159)

Italian-Style Baked Tofu
(See recipe, page 160)

Kashi Chili
(See recipe, page 161)

Lentil Vegetable Medley
(See recipe, page 162)

Rozie's Portobello Mushroom Burgers
(See recipe, page 122)

Sloppy "Toes"
(See recipe, page 123)

Spaghetti Squash with Roasted Vegetables

Squash, anyone? When spaghetti squash is cooked, the pale gold flesh turns into long, thin strands that resemble pasta. (Other varieties of squash don't work in this recipe.) Enjoy this fiber-packed delight for dinner tonight.

Spring Mix Vegetable Medley (page 224)
1 large spaghetti squash (about 3 to 4 lb/1.5 kg)
Salt and freshly ground black pepper
3 cups tomato sauce (preferably low-sodium)
Grated Parmesan cheese (optional)

1. Prepare the Spring Mix Vegetable Medley as directed, using whatever vegetables are in season.
2. Pierce the spaghetti squash all over with the point of a sharp knife. Microwave, uncovered, on high, allowing about 5 minutes per pound. Turn the squash over halfway through the cooking process. An average squash cooks in about 15 to 18 minutes in the microwave. Let stand for 5 to 10 minutes.
3. Cut the squash in half. Using a spoon or melon baller, scrape out and discard the seeds and stringy fibers. With a fork, gently separate the cooked squash into spaghetti-like strands. Discard the shells. Season the squash with salt and pepper to taste.
4. Arrange a bed of cooked spaghetti squash on each serving plate. Top with tomato sauce and reserved roasted vegetables. Reheat briefly in the microwave before serving. Sprinkle with Parmesan cheese, if desired.

Yield: 6 servings. Keeps for up to 2 days in the refrigerator; reheats well. Don't freeze.

218 calories per serving, 36.2 g carbohydrate, 8.4 g fiber, 6 g protein, 8.2 g fat (1.2 g saturated), 0 mg cholesterol, 518 mg sodium, 1197 mg potassium, 3 mg iron, 101 mg calcium

Chef's Secrets

- *What's in Store:* Although spaghetti squash is considered a winter squash, it's available year-round. The peak season is early fall through winter. It has a smooth yellow skin and looks like an overgrown football. Store spaghetti squash in a cool, dark place for up to a month.
- *Oven-Baked Squash*: Pierce the squash all over with a sharp knife so steam can escape while it cooks. Place on a baking sheet and bake, uncovered, at 400°F for about 1-¼ hours. When done, a skewer will glide easily through the flesh.
- *Sauce It Up!* Instead of commercial tomato sauce, make your own. Use Quick 'n' Easy Tomato Sauce (page 284).
- *Pest-Oh!* For a luscious, "smart-carb" dish, toss spaghetti squash with Best-O Pesto (page 282) instead of tomato sauce.
- *Say Cheese!* Instead of Parmesan cheese, use grated low-fat mozzarella, cheddar, or havarti cheese.

Sweet Potato, Cauliflower and Bean Tagine

This hearty and colorful vegetable stew is based on a recipe from Dianne Gold of Toronto. Although this Moroccan-style dish is usually served over couscous, it's also scrumptious over quinoa, barley, or wheat berries.

3 medium sweet potatoes
4 cups bite-sized cauliflower florets
2 tbsp olive oil
2 medium onions, chopped
1 red or green pepper, seeded and chopped
3 cloves garlic (about 1 tbsp minced)
1 can (19 oz/540 ml) white kidney beans, drained and rinsed
1 tsp salt (or to taste)
¼ tsp freshly ground black pepper
1 tsp ground cumin
1 tsp paprika

½ tsp ground cinnamon
¼ tsp cayenne pepper (or to taste)
3 cups tomato juice
2 cups frozen green peas (optional)
Minced fresh cilantro, for garnish

1. Pierce the sweet potatoes in several places with a sharp knife. Microwave, uncovered, on high for 8 to 10 minutes or until done but still firm. Cool slightly, then peel and cut into 1-inch chunks.
2. Rinse the cauliflower florets well but don't dry. Microwave in a covered casserole for 3 minutes on high or until nearly tender.
3. Heat the oil in a large pot on medium heat. Add the onions, red pepper, and garlic. Sauté for 2 to 3 minutes or until softened. Add the beans, reserved sweet potatoes, and cauliflower. Cook for 2 to 3 minutes longer, stirring often. Add the seasonings and tomato juice. Cover and simmer for 15 to 20 minutes or until the vegetables are tender. Stir in the frozen peas, if using. Adjust the seasonings and garnish with the minced cilantro before serving.

Yield: 10 servings of 1 cup each. Keeps for up to 3 to 4 days in the refrigerator; reheats well. Don't freeze: the vegetables will become mushy if frozen.

156 calories per serving, 27.4 g carbohydrate, 3.2 g fiber, 6 g protein, 3.2 g fat (0.5 g saturated), 0 mg cholesterol, 611 mg sodium, 694 mg potassium, 3 mg iron, 77 mg calcium

Variations
*   Substitute broccoli florets for the cauliflower, and chickpeas for the kidney beans. Instead of tomato juice, use vegetable juice or vegetable broth.
*   To boost the protein content, add 2 cups cubed extra-firm tofu, or cubed leftover cooked chicken, during the last few minutes of cooking.

Terrific Tofu Stir-Fry
(See recipe, page 167)

Vegetarian Cabbage Rolls
(See recipe, page 168)

Vegetarian Shepherd's Pie

The shepherd will be out of work if too many people discover this meatless version of shepherd's pie! This fiber-packed dish looks and tastes as if it was made with meat. Can you pull the wool over everyone's eyes?

Topping:
5 to 6 medium Yukon Gold potatoes, well-scrubbed
½ cup vegetable broth or soymilk
2 tsp extra virgin olive oil
2 tbsp low-fat or imitation sour cream
Salt and freshly ground black pepper
Paprika, for garnish

Filling:
1 tbsp olive oil
1 medium onion, chopped
1 red pepper, seeded and chopped
2 cups chopped mushrooms, or chopped zucchini
2 cloves garlic (about 2 tsp minced)
2 pkg (12 oz/340 g each) vegetarian ground beef substitute
⅓ cup tomato or barbecue sauce
1 cup corn kernels (frozen or canned)

1. In a medium saucepan, add the potatoes along with enough water to cover by 1 inch. Bring to a boil and continue boiling for about 25 minutes or until the potatoes are tender. Drain the potatoes well in a

298

strainer, then return them to the pan and dry over medium heat for 1 minute. Transfer the dried potatoes to a medium bowl and mash well. Add the broth, olive oil, sour cream, salt, and pepper to the mashed potatoes; mix well and set aside.

2. Heat the oil in a large, deep nonstick skillet on medium high. Add the onion, red pepper, mushrooms, and garlic; sauté for 5 minutes or until the onion is soft and the garlic is golden. Stir in the ground beef substitute and tomato sauce. Cook, uncovered, for 3 or 4 minutes on medium high, until heated through.

3. Remove the mixture from the skillet and transfer it to a sprayed, 2-quart rectangular casserole dish. Spread evenly. Add a layer of corn kernels, then top with a layer of the reserved potato mixture. Sprinkle with paprika. (If desired, the recipe can be assembled in advance up to this point and refrigerated overnight.)

4. Bake, uncovered, in a preheated 350°F oven for 25 to 35 minutes or until the layers are heated through and the top is golden.

Yield: 6 servings. Keeps for up to 2 to 3 days in the refrigerator; reheats well. Freezes well for up to 2 months.

332 calories per serving, 46.7 g carbohydrate, 10.7 g fiber, 25 g protein, 4.9 g fat (0.9 g saturated), 2 mg cholesterol, 693 mg sodium, 1135 mg potassium, 7 mg iron, 113 mg calcium

Nutrition Note

- *Salt Alert!* If you have sodium concerns, choose a low-sodium brand of vegetable broth and tomato sauce—or make your own. Use frozen corn kernels instead of canned.

Vegetarian Stuffed Peppers
(See recipe, page 170)

Winter Vegetable Stew
(See recipe, page 171)

Zucchini "Pasta"

This calcium-rich dish is a wonderful low-carb alternative to pasta. It's fabulous with fish and also makes a protein-packed dish if you have vegetarians at your table.

> 4 to 6 small-to-medium zucchini (about 1-½ lb/750 g), ends trimmed
> 2 cups tomato sauce (bottled or homemade)
> 1 cup grated low-fat mozzarella or Parmesan cheese

1. Cut the zucchini into pieces small enough to fit through the food processor's feed tube horizontally. (Feeding it in horizontally will produce longer shreds of zucchini.) Insert the grater into the food processor and grate the zucchini using medium pressure on the pusher. (If you have the time, you can make "fettuccine" by using a vegetable peeler to cut the zucchini into lengthwise strips.)
2. Bring a large saucepan of salted water to a boil. Add the zucchini shreds or strips to the boiling water and cook for 2 minutes, stirring 2 or 3 times, just until tender. Drain well and transfer to a platter.
3. In a small saucepan, heat the tomato sauce and pour it over the cooked zucchini. Sprinkle with cheese and serve immediately.

Yield: 4 servings. Keeps for up to 2 days in the refrigerator; reheats well in the microwave. Don't freeze.

125 calories per serving, 14.5 g carbohydrate, 4 g fiber, 10 g protein, 4.6 g fat (2.9 g saturated), 16 mg cholesterol, 776 mg sodium, 390 mg potassium, 1 mg iron, 206 mg calcium

CHAPTER SEVEN

DESSERT

WHAT'S INSIDE

■ CHILLED OR FROZEN DESSERTS

The fruit in many frozen desserts boosts the fiber—and the flavor!

Apple Blue-Peary Sauce
(See recipe, page 32)

Berry Fool

A fool is a creamy dessert traditionally made with whipped cream and fruit. This light, calcium-packed version tastes decadent, but you can enjoy it without the guilt (no fooling)! Drained yogurt replaces the whipped cream. Feel free to use any soft-textured, ripe berries or fruit such as peaches, nectarines, or bananas.

> 3 cups nonfat plain natural yogurt (without gelatin or stabilizers)
> 3 cups whole strawberries (hulled), raspberries, or blackberries
> 3 to 4 tbsp granulated sugar, maple syrup, or granular Splenda

1. Line a fine mesh strainer with a paper coffee filter, a paper towel, or cheese-cloth. Place the lined strainer over a glass bowl or large measuring cup. Spoon the yogurt into the lined strainer, cover, and refrigerate. Let drain for 2 hours. When done, you'll have 2 cups of thick yogurt in the strainer and 1 cup of liquid whey in the bowl. Discard the liquid whey or store it in the refrigerator, covered, and use in recipes as a substitute for buttermilk.
2. Set aside 1 cup of the berries. (If using strawberries, thinly slice 1 cup and set aside.) In a food processor fitted with the steel blade, process the remaining berries until puréed, about 15 to 20 seconds. Add the drained yogurt and the sugar; process with several quick on/off pulses, just until combined.
3. Pour half the mixture into four parfait glasses, and then top with a layer of the reserved berries. Repeat with the remaining mixture and another layer of berries. Chill for at least 1 to 2 hours before serving.

Yield: 4 servings. Keeps for up to 2 days in the refrigerator. Don't freeze.

151 calories per serving, 33.2 g carbohydrate, 2.5 g fiber, 8 g protein, 0.4 g fat (0 g satu-rated), 4 mg cholesterol, 102 mg sodium, 191 mg potassium, 1 mg iron, 245 mg calcium With Splenda, one serving contains 119 calories and 24.9 g carbohydrate.

Variation
- **Mango Fool:** Instead of strawberries, substitute 3 peeled and pitted mangoes. Slice 1 mango and set aside; purée the remaining two. Prepare as directed above.

Chef's Secrets
- *Whey to Go!* Save the drained liquid (whey) and use it instead of butter-milk when baking muffins and cakes. It will keep up to 2 weeks in the refrigerator.
- *Measure Up:* To measure how much yogurt you've got after draining, measure the drained whey. Three cups of yogurt yield 1 cup of whey and 2 cups of drained yogurt. If the drained yogurt is too firm, don't worry. Just stir some of the whey back in.

Berry Mango Sherbet
Keep frozen fruit on hand in your freezer so you can make this guilt-free dessert in moments. It's "berry" refreshing—great for friends and family!

3 cups frozen strawberries, blueberries, and/or raspberries
1 cup frozen mango chunks
¼–⅓ cup granulated sugar or granular Splenda
1 cup plain yogurt (nonfat or low-fat)

1. In a food processor fitted with the steel blade, process the frozen berries, mango, and sugar with several quick on/off pulses. Continue running the motor until the mixture has the texture of snow. Add the yogurt and process until very smooth, scraping down the sides of the bowl as needed.

2. Serve immediately in parfait glasses or transfer to a bowl, cover, and freeze. About 30 minutes before serving, remove from the freezer and place in the refrigerator to soften. Scoop into parfait or wine glasses and serve.

Yield: About 4 cups (6 servings of ⅔ cup each).

90 calories per serving, 21.8 g carbohydrate, 2.5 g fiber, 2 g protein, 0.1 g fat (0 g saturated), 1 mg cholesterol, 23 mg sodium, 43 mg potassium, 0 mg iron, 63 mg calcium. If you use Splenda instead of sugar, one serving contains 74 calories and 16.8 g carbohydrate.

Chef's Secrets
- *Mix It Up!* You can create different flavors by using a total of 4 cups frozen mixed fruit.
- *Berry Easy!* To make a small batch, use 1 cup frozen fruit, 1 tbsp granulated sugar or Splenda, and ¼ cup yogurt.

Chocolate Tofu Mousse

Cocoa and tofu make for a delicious pairing, and they have more in common than you'd think. Both come from beans (cocoa beans and soybeans), both are relatively healthy, and both are scrumptious in desserts. So, if you can keep a secret, no one will ever guess this luscious dessert has anything to do with tofu, unless of course you tell them!

1 pkg (16 oz/500 g) extra-firm or firm silken tofu, well-drained
¾ cup granular Splenda or granulated sugar
⅔ cup unsweetened cocoa powder
1 tsp pure vanilla or almond extract
Frozen light whipped topping and grated semi-sweet chocolate, for garnish

1. In a food processor fitted with the steel blade, process the tofu for 1 to 2 minutes or until very smooth. Scrape down the sides of the bowl as needed. Add Splenda, cocoa, and vanilla and process until blended, about 20 seconds longer.

2. Transfer the mixture into four parfait or wine glasses; garnish with whipped topping and grated chocolate. Chill for 1 to 2 hours, or until serving time.

Yield: 4 servings. Keeps for up to 2 to 3 days in the refrigerator. Don't freeze.

96 calories per serving, 13.6 g carbohydrate, 4.3 g fiber, 11 g protein, 2.7 g fat (1.2 g saturated), 0 mg cholesterol, 114 mg sodium, 426 mg potassium, 3 mg iron, 65 mg calcium. Sweet Choice—If you use sugar instead of Splenda, one serving contains 168 calories and 36.1 g carbohydrate.

Chef's Secrets

- *Doubly Delicious:* Some brands of silken tofu come in a 12-oz/340-g package. Use 2 packages and make 1-½ times the recipe (6 servings). You'll be glad you did!
- *Smooth as Silk:* Silken tofu is dairy-free, cholesterol-free, and silky smooth. It provides a wonderful creamy texture that's creamier than cream itself! You can use it instead of whipped cream or whipped dessert topping in desserts.

Frozen Peanut Butter Mousse

This sugar-free dessert tastes like ice cream. However, even though there's no added sugar, it's still quite high in calories and saturated fat because of the peanut butter, so save it for special occasions.

    1 cup 1% cottage cheese or light cream cheese
    1 cup natural peanut butter
    ¾ cup granular Splenda
    2 cups frozen light whipped topping, thawed
    1 tsp pure vanilla extract

1. In a food processor fitted with the steel blade, process the cottage cheese until smooth and creamy, about 2 minutes, scraping down the sides of the bowl as needed.

305

2. Add the peanut butter, Splenda, whipped topping, and vanilla; process until well blended, about 25 to 30 seconds. Divide the mixture into individual serving dishes; cover and freeze.

Yield: 8 servings. Freezes well for up to 1 month.

271 calories per serving, 16.1 g carbohydrate, 2 g fiber, 11 g protein, 18.3 g fat (4.2 g saturated), 1 mg cholesterol, 235 mg sodium, 25 mg potassium, 0 mg iron, 17 mg calcium. Sweet Choice—If you use sugar instead of Splenda, one serving contains 334 calories and 32.6 g carbohydrate.

Dairy-Free Variation

- Replace the cream cheese with Tofutti imitation cream cheese and instead of light whipped topping, use non-dairy topping that has been whipped in an electric mixer until stiff.

Luscious Lemon Berry Mousse

Picture perfect! This creamy, lemony dessert is like trifle without the cake. The best time to make this dessert is in the summertime, when fresh berries are plentiful and inexpensive. Your guests will think it's so decadent.

1 pkg (7-½ oz/212 g) lemon pie filling (the kind you cook)
1-½ cups softened fat-free or light cream cheese
3 cups frozen light whipped topping, thawed
3 cups fresh blueberries
2 cups raspberries or strawberries, hulled and halved

1. Prepare the pie filling according to the package directions. (To microwave the filling, cook on high in an 8-cup glass batter bowl for 3 to 4 minutes, stirring once or twice, until bubbly and thick.) Cool for 5 to 10 minutes.
2. Add the cream cheese, by heaping tablespoonfuls, to the hot lemon mixture, whisking well after each addition. Continue whisking until smooth and blended. Cover and refrigerate for 1 hour.

3.   When the mixture is fully chilled, whisk in the whipped topping. Pour ⅓ of the lemon mixture into a large glass serving bowl and layer with half the blueberries. Add another ⅓ of the lemon mixture and layer with most of the raspberries. Top with the remaining lemon mixture and arrange the remaining blueberries around the edge of the bowl and the raspberries in the center. Cover and store in the refrigerator overnight. Serve chilled.

Yield: 12 servings. Keeps for up to 2 to 3 days in the refrigerator. Don't freeze.

161 calories per serving, 28.1 g carbohydrate, 2.3 g fiber, 6 g protein, 3.7 g fat (2.6 g saturated), 26 mg cholesterol, 182 mg sodium, 97 mg potassium, 0 mg iron, 63 mg calcium

Chef's Secret

- *How Light?* This recipe can also be made with light cream cheese, but the saturated fat content is significantly higher. One serving contains 204 calories and 8.3 g fat (5.8 g saturated).

Mock Banana Soft Ice Cream

2 large ripe bananas, sliced
½ cup nonfat cottage cheese or part-skim ricotta cheese
½ tsp vanilla
4 tsp sugar

1.   Arrange banana slices in a single layer on a waxed-paper lined plate. Cover and freeze until firm. Frozen slices can be frozen in a tightly sealed container for up to a month. (I've also frozen whole bananas in their skins, then removed them from the freezer at serving time and placed them under running water for 30 seconds. Peel with a sharp knife and cut into chunks.) At serving time, combine ingredients in the processor and process until smooth. Serve immediately.

Yield: 4 servings.

102 calories per serving, 0.3 g fat (0.1 g saturated), 3 mg cholesterol, 5 g protein, 22 g carbohydrate, 93 mg sodium, 300 mg potassium, trace iron, 2 g fiber, 19 mg calcium

Variations

- **Mock Banana-Strawberry Soft Ice Cream:** Follow the recipe above, using 1 banana and 1-½ cups ripe strawberries. One serving contains 82 calories and 16 g carbohydrate.
- **Easiest Frozen Banana Mousse:** Peel and slice 4 ripe bananas. Arrange in a single layer on a plate and cover tightly to prevent them from absorbing any odors. Freeze completely. When needed, thaw for 5 minutes, then process with 1 teaspoon of lemon juice in the processor until smooth. Serve immediately. Makes 4 servings.

Pumpkin Cheesecake

This scrumptious pumpkin cheesecake can be made lighter by using half cream cheese and half cottage cheese. Or you can make it dairy-free by using imitation cream cheese. It's perfect for Thanksgiving—your guests will be so thankful!

Crust:
1 cup graham wafer crumbs
2 tbsp canola oil
1 tbsp brown sugar or granular Splenda

Filling:
3 cups (1-½ lb/750 g) light cream cheese or imitation cream cheese such as Tofutti
1 cup granulated sugar or granular Splenda
1 cup canned pumpkin
3 eggs (or ¾ cup liquid eggs)
1 tsp pure vanilla extract
1 tsp pumpkin pie spice

1. Preheat the oven to 350°F. Spray a 9-inch springform pan with cooking spray. Place a pie plate, half-filled with water, on the lowest rack of the oven. (This helps prevent the cheesecake from cracking.)
2. *Crust:* Combine the crumbs with the oil and brown sugar in a bowl; mix well. Pat into the bottom of the prepared pan.
3. *Filling:* In a food processor fitted with the steel blade, process the cream cheese, sugar, and pumpkin until blended, about 20 seconds. Add the eggs, vanilla, and pumpkin pie spice; process until smooth and creamy, 20 to 30 seconds longer. Pour over crust.
4. Place the cheesecake on the middle rack. Bake for 40 to 45 minutes. When done, the edges will be set, but the center will jiggle slightly.
5. Turn off the heat and let the cheesecake cool in the oven with the door partly open for 1 hour. The cheesecake will firm up during this time. Remove the cheesecake from the oven and let cool. Cover and refrigerate overnight, or for up to 2 days. When ready to serve, remove the sides of the pan from the chilled cheesecake and transfer to a serving plate.

Yield: 12 servings. Keeps for up to 2 to 3 days in the refrigerator. Don't freeze: if frozen, the crust will become soggy.

275 calories per serving, 28.6 g carbohydrate, 0.8 g fiber, 8 g protein, 14.3 g fat (7.1 g saturated), 85 mg cholesterol, 229 mg sodium, 167 mg potassium, 2 mg iron, 79 mg calcium. If you use Splenda instead of sugar, one serving contains 216 calories and 13.4 g carbohydrate.

Chef's Secrets

- *No pumpkin pie spice?* Combine ½ tsp ground cinnamon, ¼ tsp ground nutmeg, and ¼ tsp ground allspice.
- *Top It Up!* If your cheesecake develops cracks in the top during baking, don't worry. Combine 1 cup light sour cream, 2 tbsp granulated sugar or Splenda, and 1 tsp pure vanilla extract; mix well. Pour carefully on top of the cheesecake and bake 6 to 8 minutes longer. Topping will firm up when chilled.

Dairy-Free Variation
- Make the cheesecake with imitation cream cheese. Brush the top of the baked cheesecake with ¼ cup melted apricot preserves and sprinkle with ½ cup toasted sliced almonds. It will taste just like regular cheesecake.

Strawberry and Banana Frozen Yogurt
For maximum flavor, use very ripe fruit for this recipe.

> 1 pint very ripe strawberries, hulled (or 2 cups unsweetened frozen berries)
> 3 very ripe medium bananas, peeled
> ½ cup nonfat yogurt
> 1 to 2 tbsp honey (to taste)

1. Cut fruit into 1-inch pieces. Arrange in a single layer on a baking sheet and freeze for 2 or 3 hours, until firm. (Fruit can be frozen for several weeks in plastic storage bags.)
2. Place the processor bowl and steel knife into the freezer for 15 to 20 minutes. Combine all ingredients in chilled processor bowl. Process with quick on/offs to start, then let machine run until mixture is smooth. (If you have a small processor, do this in 2 batches.) Serve immediately, or transfer mixture to a serving bowl and freeze for up to ½ hour before serving.

Yield: 6 servings.

91 calories per serving, 0.5 g fat (0.1 g saturated), trace cholesterol, 2 g protein, 22 g carbohydrate, 17 mg sodium, 371 mg potassium, trace iron, 3 g fiber, 52 mg calcium

Strawberry Buttermilk Sherbet

So pretty, so delicious! Leftover buttermilk can be used in muffin or cake recipes.

1-½–2 cups frozen strawberries
¼ cup sugar or honey
¼–⅓ cup buttermilk
1 tsp lemon juice

1. Process berries with sugar until the texture of snow. Gradually add buttermilk and lemon juice through the feed tube. Process until well mixed and the texture of sherbet. Serve immediately.

Yield: 3 to 4 servings. Recipe can be doubled easily.

99 calories per serving, 0.3 g fat (0.1 g saturated), <1 mg cholesterol, 1 g protein, 25 g carbohydrate, 23 mg sodium, 144 mg potassium, <1 mg iron, 2 g fiber, 36 mg calcium

Variations
- Either use 1 package of frozen unsweetened strawberries (about 1-½ cups), or freeze 2 cups of very ripe strawberries for this recipe. The more berries you use, the more buttermilk you need to add.
- Raspberries can be used instead of strawberries. Nonfat yogurt can be used instead of buttermilk.

Strawberry Kiwi Parfaits

Love that layered look! These colorful, fiber-filled parfaits are perfect for company.

1 cup fat-free or low-fat cottage cheese
1 cup nonfat or low-fat plain yogurt
3 tbsp granulated sugar or granular Splenda
½ tsp pure vanilla extract
4 cups strawberries, hulled and sliced
4 kiwifruit, peeled and diced
6 whole strawberries, for garnish

1. In a food processor fitted with the steel blade, combine the cottage cheese, yogurt, sugar, vanilla, and 2 cups of strawberries. Process until very smooth, scraping down the sides of the bowl as needed.
2. Layer the remaining sliced strawberries in the bottom of four parfait glasses. Follow with a layer of half the cheese mixture, a layer of kiwifruit, then the remaining cheese mixture. Top each parfait with a whole strawberry. Cover and refrigerate for 1 to 2 hours, or until well chilled.

Yield: 6 servings. Recipe doubles or triples easily. Keeps in the refrigerator for a day or two. Don't freeze.

144 calories per serving, 29.4 g carbohydrate, 4.1 g fiber, 7 g protein, 0.6 g fat (0 g saturated), 4 mg cholesterol, 175 mg sodium, 356 mg potassium, 1 mg iron, 115 mg calcium. Sweet Choice—If you use granular Splenda instead of sugar, one serving contains 123 calories and 23.9 g carbohydrate.

Nutrition Notes
- Kiwifruit (GI 53) is high in vision-saving lutein, vitamin C, and fiber. It is a good source of vitamin E and potassium.
- Strawberries (GI 40) are high in vitamin C, potassium, fiber, folate, and antioxidants. Too many can have a diuretic and laxative effect.

■ FRUIT DESSERTS

Fruit makes an easy high fiber dessert. Plain fruit in season, or a fruit salad, is always a welcome, light dessert. Or dress it up in the following recipes.

Fabulous Fruit Crisp
(See recipe, page 63)

Jumbleberry Crisp
(See recipe, page 65)

Madeleine's Fruit Clafouti
(See recipe, page 66)

Melons and Berries in Wine
A light and refreshing dessert, loaded with potassium and fiber.

1-½ cups medium white wine
2 tbsp honey or sugar
2–3 slices ginger root
½ of a medium cantaloupe, halved and seeded
½ of a honeydew, seeded
½ of a Casaba or Crenshaw melon, seeded
2 cups fresh strawberries, hulled and halved
1–2 cups fresh blueberries

1. In a saucepan, combine wine with honey and ginger. Bring to a boil, reduce heat and simmer uncovered for 5 minutes. Remove from heat and let cool to room temperature. Discard ginger.
2. Use a melon baller to scoop out balls from the melons. Place in a large bowl along with the strawberries and blueberries. Pour the cooled wine over fruit and mix gently. Refrigerate for 1 to 2 hours to blend the flavors. Spoon fruit into chilled serving dishes. Drizzle wine over fruit.

Yield: 8 servings.

162 calories per serving, 0.6 g fat (0.1 g saturated), 0 mg cholesterol, 3 g protein, 33 g carbohydrate, 40 mg sodium, 876 mg potassium, 1 mg iron, 4 g fiber, 30 mg calcium

Variations
- **Super Smoothie:** Combine the flesh of ½ cantaloupe, ½ melon, 1 banana, 8 strawberries, and a few ice cubes in the blender or processor. Makes 2 servings.

- Half a cantaloupe supplies nearly double the daily recommended intake of vitamin C. It will provide as much vitamin C as 1-½ oranges. Cantaloupe is also a great source of beta carotene. So save the other half of the cantaloupe for a mega-healthy breakfast. The vitamin C in the melon enhances iron absorption from your bowl of cereal.

Peachy Crumb Crisp
(See recipe, page 67)

Poached Pears
Juicy fruit! Pears take on a lovely rosy hue from the cooking juices in this easy, elegant dessert.

> 1 cup cranberry juice (low-calorie or regular)
> 1 cinnamon stick or ¼ tsp ground cinnamon
> 1 tbsp honey
> 1 tsp lemon juice (preferably fresh)
> 4 firm ripe pears such as Bosc or Anjou

1. Combine the cranberry juice, cinnamon, honey, and lemon juice in a large skillet over high heat; bring to a boil. Reduce heat to low and simmer for 2 minutes.
2. Peel the pears and cut in half lengthwise. Remove the cores with a melon baller. Place, cut-side down, in the skillet, with the narrow ends pointing inward.
3. Cover and continue simmering for 8 to 10 minutes, basting occasionally. When done, the pears should hold their shape but be tender and easily pierced with a knife. Serve warm or chilled, with the sauce spooned over the pears.

Yield: 4 servings. Keeps for up to 3 to 4 days in the refrigerator. Don't freeze.

109 calories per serving, 28.9 g carbohydrate, 4.5 g fiber, 1 g protein, 0.2 g fat (0 g saturated), 0 mg cholesterol, 5 mg sodium, 197 mg potassium, 1 mg iron, 21 mg calcium

Chef's Secrets

- *Wing It!* Place 2 poached pear halves on each dessert dish, with their stem ends touching. Slice each half lengthwise, from the wide end to just past the middle, so that each sliced piece is still attached at the narrow end. Fan out the sliced ends; you will have an appealing butterfly design.
- *"Nut"-ritious:* At serving time, sprinkle the poached pears with toasted slivered almonds.
- *Juice It Up!* Instead of cranberry juice, use pomegranate juice and increase the amount of honey to 2 tbsp. Other juice options to consider are apple-raspberry, cranberry-orange, cran-raspberry, or cran-blueberry juice. Juggle your juices!
- *Leftovers?* Slice any leftover pears and combine with your favorite flavor of nonfat yogurt for breakfast. Or serve pears with vanilla frozen yogurt for dessert—a drizzle of chocolate couldn't hurt!

Simply Ambrosia

10 oz (285 ml) can pineapple tidbits, drained
3 large seedless oranges, peeled and cut in ½-inch chunks
1 cup seedless grapes
2 cups strawberries, halved
3 cups miniature marshmallows
3 cups low-fat lemon yogurt
6 chocolate cookies, crushed

1. Pat fruit dry. Combine fruit, marshmallows, and yogurt in a bowl; mix gently. Transfer to a glass serving bowl and sprinkle with cookie crumbs. Cover and chill overnight.

Yield: 12 servings.

149 calories per serving, 1.5 g fat (0.6 g saturated), 3 mg cholesterol, 5 g protein, 32 g carbohydrate, 64 mg sodium, 327 mg potassium, <1 mg iron, 2 g fiber, 134 mg calcium

Citrus or Melon Baskets

- *Basket without Handle:* Trim top and bottom of citrus fruit or melon to form a stable base at both ends. Cut in half with a V-shaped knife (or make uniform zigzag cuts with a sharp knife), cutting all the way through to the center. Adjust the last cut to meet the first cut. Separate the halves. Use a melon baller to hollow out melon. Pulp from citrus fruit can be removed with a sharp paring knife or grapefruit knife. Fill grapefruit, orange, or melon baskets with colorful fresh fruit salad.
- *Basket with Handle:* Trim bottom of fruit to form a stable base. Cut away two wedges from the top side so you are left with a handle in the middle of the basket. Make uniform zigzag cuts around basket and handle with a V-shaped or sharp knife, adjusting the last cut to meet the first cut. (Don't cut through the handle!) Cut away pulp under the handle with a sharp knife. Remove pulp, leaving a shell that is firm enough to hold the filling. Use a small ice cream scoop for watermelon, a melon baller for smaller melons, and a grapefruit knife for citrus fruit. A few hours in advance, fill as desired. Trim the handle with overlapping citrus slices anchored with toothpicks. Top each toothpick with a grape or strawberry. Refrigerate until serving time.

Strawberries with Balsamic Vinegar or Red Wine

The natural sugars in the berries and vinegar make a yummy syrup. Always rinse berries before you remove the stems. Otherwise, berries will become waterlogged.

2 pints strawberries
1 tbsp orange juice or Grand Marnier
3 tbsp balsamic vinegar or red wine
3 tbsp brown sugar (or to taste)

1. Rinse, hull, and slice berries. Mix gently with remaining ingredients. Refrigerate covered for at least ½ hour. (The longer they stand, the more delicious they become.)

Yield: 4 to 6 servings.

94 calories per serving, 0.6 g fat (0 g saturated), 0 mg cholesterol, 1 g protein, 23 g carbohydrate, 8 mg sodium, 283 mg potassium, <1 mg iron, 3 g fiber, 31 mg calcium

Strawberry Surprise

One cup of strawberries contains 85 mg of vitamin C, more than an orange! Strawberries are packed with antioxidants and contain virtually no fat. One cup of berries contains 46 calories and more than 3 grams of fiber. Now that's very berry good news, and so are the desserts that follow!

3 cups nonfat natural yogurt (without gelatin or stabilizers)
4 cups ripe strawberries, hulled and sliced
2–3 tbsp orange liqueur (e.g., Sabra)
3 tbsp maple syrup or honey (to taste)

1. Line a strainer with a paper coffee filter, paper toweling, or a cheesecloth. Place strainer over a large glass measuring cup or bowl. Spoon yogurt into strainer and let drain for 1 hour, or until yogurt has reduced to 2 cups. (Drained whey can be used instead of buttermilk or yogurt in baking.)
2. Sprinkle strawberries with liqueur and marinate for 30 minutes; drain. Fold half of berries into thickened yogurt. Sweeten to taste. Layer remaining berries and yogurt mixture in 6 parfait or wine glasses, starting and ending with berries. Chill before serving.

Yield: 6 servings. Leftovers can be refrigerated for up to 2 days if well-covered.

131 calories per serving, 0.6 g fat (0.1 g saturated), 2 mg cholesterol, 7 g protein, 24 g carbohydrate, 60 mg sodium, 382 mg potassium, trace iron, 2 g fiber, 171 mg calcium

Variations

- If you don't have any orange liqueur on hand, substitute 2 tablespoons of white wine and 1 tablespoon orange juice. If desired, arrange a layer of peeled, sliced kiwis as the middle layer.

- **Strawberry Pudding Parfaits:** Instead of yogurt, substitute 1 pkg (6 serving size) vanilla pudding mix. Cook according to package directions, using skim milk. Stir 1 tablespoon of orange liqueur into cooked pudding. Cover to prevent a skin from forming; chill. Layer marinated strawberries and pudding in parfait glasses. Chill before serving.
- **Strawberry and Ice Cream Parfaits:** Instead of drained yogurt, substitute low-fat ice cream (strawberry or vanilla) or frozen yogurt. Layer marinated strawberries and ice cream in parfait glasses. Serve immediately. (This is also scrumptious if you prepare the yogurt/berry mixture as directed in the main recipe and use it as a topping over the ice cream and strawberries!)

■ COOKIES

Loaded with oats, raisins, and nuts, cookies can be packed with fiber. But usually with fat and sugar, too, so count your cookies!

Best Oatmeal Cookies

These scrumptious cookies are a new twist on an old favorite. They're "oat" of this world! For dairy-free cookies, choose a brand of chocolate chips that contain no dairy products.

½ cup canola oil
2 egg whites (or 1 large egg)
⅓ cup lightly packed brown sugar
⅓ cup granulated sugar
2 tbsp water
1 tsp pure vanilla extract
¾ cup whole-wheat flour
1-½ cups rolled oats (preferably large flake)
¼ cup wheat germ
½ tsp baking soda
1 tsp ground cinnamon

⅛ tsp salt
⅓ cup semi-sweet chocolate chips
⅓ cup raisins or dried cranberries
⅓ cup sunflower seeds or chopped almonds, walnuts, or pecans (optional)

1. Place the oven rack in the middle of the oven and preheat to 350°F. Line two large baking sheets with parchment paper.
2. In a food processor fitted with the steel blade (or in a large bowl and using an electric mixer), beat the oil, egg whites, sugars, water, and vanilla until well-blended, about 1 minute. Add the flour, rolled oats, wheat germ, baking soda, cinnamon, and salt; mix well. If using a food processor, transfer the batter to a large bowl. Stir in the chocolate chips, raisins, and seeds or nuts.
3. Drop the batter from a teaspoon onto the prepared baking sheets. Bake for 10 to 12 minutes or until golden.

Yield: About 3-½ dozen cookies. Store in a covered container. Freezes well for up to 4 months.

66 calories per cookie, 8.3 g carbohydrate, 0.8 g fiber, 1 g protein, 3.4 g fat (0.5 g saturated), 0 mg cholesterol, 26 mg sodium, 46 mg potassium, 0 mg iron, 5 mg calcium

Nutrition Notes

- Wheat germ or wheat bran—what's the difference? They're separate parts of the same grain: the bran is the outer coating and the wheat germ is the inner part. Wheat germ supplies nutrients such as protein, B vitamins, and vitamin E, whereas wheat bran has more fiber. So include both in your diet for good health.

Brownie Cookies

Instead of baking brownies in a baking pan, drop them, by teaspoonfuls, onto a cookie sheet. These crispy cookies are flatter but larger in diameter than square-cut brownies, so you get more bites for the same number of calories. You'll definitely get brownie points for making these!

¼ cup soft tub margarine
¼ cup unsweetened applesauce
½ cup granulated sugar
½ cup lightly packed brown sugar
2 large eggs (or 1 large egg plus 2 egg whites)
1 tsp pure vanilla extract
¾ cup whole-wheat flour
½ cup unsweetened cocoa powder
½ tsp baking powder
⅛ tsp salt
25 walnut or pecan halves

1. Preheat the oven to 350°F. Line a baking sheet with parchment paper.
2. In a food processor fitted with the steel blade, combine the margarine, applesauce, sugars, eggs, and vanilla; process for 1 minute or until well-blended. Add the flour, cocoa, baking powder, and salt; process with several quick on/off pulses, just until blended. Don't overprocess.
3. Drop the batter from a tablespoon onto the prepared baking sheet, leaving 3 inches between each mound. Place a walnut on top of each mound.
4. Bake for 13 to 15 minutes or until the tops are set when touched with your fingertips; don't overbake. Cool for 5 minutes before removing from the pan.

Yield: 25 cookies. Freezes well for up to 4 months.

78 calories per cookie/brownie, 11 g carbohydrate, 1.2 g fiber, 2 g protein, 3.7 g fat (0. 6g saturated), 8 mg cholesterol, 55 mg sodium, 70 mg potassium, 1 mg iron, 15 mg calcium

Variation

- **Brownies:** Melt the margarine, then prepare the batter as directed. Spread evenly in a sprayed, 8-inch square glass baking dish. Place the nuts 5 across and 5 down. Bake at 350°F for 25 minutes. When done, the top will be set when touched with your fingertips and a cake tester or tooth-pick inserted into the center of the cake will come out slightly moist. Don't overbake. Once cooled, cut into 25 small squares.

Chef's Secrets

- *No Nuts for You!* Without nuts, one cookie/brownie contains 65 calories, and 2.3 g fat (0.5 g saturated).
- *Kidding Around:* Instead of nuts, top each cookie/brownie with an M&M. Mmmm!
- *Super-Size Me!* If you want bigger brownies, cut them into 16 squares. One brownie with nuts contains 114 calories, 17.1 g carbohydrate, 1.8 g fiber, and 5 g fat (0.9 saturated).

Chocolate Chewies

Pretty as a picture! These are a chocoholic's delight.

½ cup unsweetened cocoa
2 cups icing sugar
2 tbsp flour
3 egg whites
½ tsp vanilla
1-¾ cups low-fat granola cereal
¼ cup finely chopped almonds or walnuts

1. Preheat oven to 350°F. Line 2 baking sheets with aluminum foil and spray with nonstick spray. In the large bowl of an electric mixer, combine cocoa, icing sugar, and flour. Blend in egg whites on low speed. Increase to high speed and beat 1 to 2 minutes longer. Stir in vanilla, cereal, and nuts.

2. Drop mixture by rounded teaspoonfuls on baking sheets, leaving about 2 inches between cookies. Press tops slightly with the bottom of a small glass to flatten. Bake on middle rack at 350°F for about 15 minutes, until set and crispy. Cool completely. Store in an airtight container.

Yield: About 4 dozen. Can be frozen.

41 calories per cookie, 0.7 g fat (0.1 g saturated), 0 mg cholesterol, <1 g protein, 9 g carbohydrate, 14 mg sodium, 33 mg potassium, trace iron, < 1 g fiber, 3 mg calcium

Chocolate Chip Cookies

Oat-so-good! This recipe comes from my favorite (and only) daughter, Jodi Sprackman, who is an excellent cook and baker. My granddaughters call them "Jodi's Oaties!" Lauren and Camille love to bake and are showing great potential as future chefs.

½ cup soft tub margarine
½ cup lightly packed brown sugar
¼ cup granulated sugar
1 large egg
1 tsp pure vanilla extract
¾ cup whole-wheat flour
½ tsp baking soda
¼ tsp salt
1-½ cups quick-cooking oats (preferably large flake)
¾ to 1 cup semi-sweet chocolate chips

1. Preheat the oven to 350°F. Line 2 large baking sheets with parchment paper.
2. In a food processor fitted with the steel blade, combine the margarine, sugars, egg, and vanilla; process for 2 minutes or until well-blended. Add the flour, baking soda, salt, and oats; process with quick on/off pulses, just until combined. Stir in the chocolate chips with a rubber spatula.

3. Drop from a teaspoon onto the prepared baking sheets, leaving 2 inches between each cookie. Bake for 12 to 15 minutes or until golden. Cool for 5 minutes, then remove from pan.

Yield: About 44 cookies. Recipe can be doubled easily. Freezes well for up to 4 months.

62 calories per cookie, 7.9 g carbohydrate, 0.7 g fiber, 1 g protein, 3.3 g fat (0.9 g saturated), 5 mg cholesterol, 58 mg sodium, 37 mg potassium, 0 mg iron, 6 mg calcium

Variations
- Use only ½ cup chocolate chips and add ½ cup chopped pecans or walnuts.
- Instead of nuts, substitute dried cherries, cranberries, or raisins.

Peanut Butter Cookies

Three ingredients, three minutes to mix up the batter, and less than three minutes before they're gone! You can make these gluten-free cookies with sugar or Splenda, but either way they might turn you into a glutton, so practice portion control and save these as an occasional treat.

> 1 cup creamy or crunchy natural peanut butter
> ¾ cup granulated sugar or granular Splenda
> 1 large egg

1. Preheat the oven to 325°F. Line a large baking sheet with parchment paper.
2. In a mixing bowl, combine the peanut butter, sugar, and egg; mix well. Drop by rounded teaspoonfuls onto the prepared baking sheet, leaving 2 inches between each cookie. (If you use Splenda, place a piece of parchment or wax paper on top of the unbaked cookies and press gently to flatten them before baking; see Chef's Secrets, page 324.) Uncover before baking.
3. Bake for 10 minutes or until cookies are golden. Remove from the oven and let cool on the baking sheet for 10 to 15 minutes. The cookies will firm up as they cool.

Yield: 26 cookies (if made with sugar) or 21 cookies (if made with Splenda). Freezes well for up to 4 months.

87 calories per cookie (with sugar), 7.9 g carbohydrate, 0.6 g fiber, 2 g protein, 5.1 g fat (0.7 g saturated), 8 mg cholesterol, 40 mg sodium, 3 mg potassium, 0 mg iron, 1 mg calcium. Sweet Choice—83 calories per cookie using Splenda, 3.5 g carbohydrate, 0.8 g fiber, 3 g protein, 6.3 g fat (0.8 g saturated), 10 mg cholesterol, 49 mg sodium, 3 mg potassium, 0 mg iron, 1 mg calcium

Chef's Secrets

- *What's the Spread?* Cookies made with sugar will spread during baking, whereas cookies made with Splenda will stay in a mound and won't spread unless you flatten them before baking.
- *Batter Up!* You get more batter (and cookies) when using sugar, but less batter (and cookies) with Splenda. That's the way the cookie crumbles!

Skinny Lemon Biscotti

These thin, crisp biscotti have a lovely lemon flavor and are packed with almonds and dried fruit. You'll go nuts over them!

4 egg whites (or 2 large eggs)
½ cup granulated sugar
2 tbsp canola oil
1 tsp pure vanilla extract
1 tbsp grated lemon rind
1 tbsp lemon juice (preferably fresh)
1 cup whole-wheat flour
½ tsp baking powder
⅔ cup slivered almonds
⅔ cup chopped dried apricots
½ tsp ground cinnamon mixed with 1 tbsp granulated sugar

1. Preheat the oven to 350°F. Spray a small (8- by 4-inch) loaf pan with cooking spray.
2. Beat the egg whites with sugar, oil, and vanilla until well mixed, about 2 minutes. Add the lemon rind, juice, flour, and baking powder. Stir in almonds and apricots and mix until combined. Pour into the prepared pan and spread evenly.
3. Bake for 30 to 35 minutes or until golden. Let cool for 10 to 15 minutes, then invert and remove the loaf from the pan. Wrap in foil and refrigerate overnight (or up to 2 days).
4. Unwrap the loaf and slice as thinly as possible, about ¼-inch thick, with a sharp serrated knife. Arrange slices in a single layer on parchment-lined baking sheet(s). Sprinkle lightly with cinnamon-sugar mixture. Bake in a preheated 250oF oven for 30 to 40 minutes, until crisp and toasted.

Yield: About 32 slices. Store in a loosely covered container. Freezes well for up to 4 months.

58 calories per slice, 8.8 g carbohydrate, 1 g fiber, 2 g protein, 2.1 g fat (0.2 g saturated), 0 mg cholesterol, 15 mg sodium, 75 mg potassium, 0 mg iron, 14 mg calcium

Variations
- Instead of almonds, substitute flaked Brazil nuts or coarsely chopped walnuts.
- Instead of dried apricots, substitute with dried cranberries or raisins.

Slimmer Hello Dollies

My dear daughter, Jodi Sprackman, adores these! I've reduced the fat substantially from the original recipe, but "Dolly" didn't say "Goodbye" to all the fat, so save them for special occasions. Low-fat sweetened condensed milk has half the fat of regular condensed milk, but almost the same calories!

⅓ cup tub margarine or butter
1-⅓ cups graham cracker crumbs
1 cup flaked or shredded coconut

⅔ cup semi-sweet chocolate chips

½ cup pecans or almonds

14 oz can (1-⅓ cups/300 ml) sweetened condensed skim milk (low-fat)

1. Preheat oven to 350°F. Spray a 9- by 13-inch pan with nonstick spray. Put margarine in pan and place in the oven to melt. Mix in crumbs and spread evenly in pan. Sprinkle with coconut. Coarsely chop chocolate chips and pecans in processor. Sprinkle over coconut. Drizzle condensed milk evenly over the top. Bake at 350°F for 25 minutes, until golden. Cool completely. Cut into squares.

Yield: 4 dozen. Freeze leftovers, but seal your mouth with masking tape until they're packed away!

81 calories per square, 4.5 g fat (1.9 g saturated), 1 mg cholesterol, 1 g protein, 10 g carbohydrate, 40 mg sodium, 57 mg potassium, trace iron, <1 g fiber, 26 mg calcium

■ CRISPS, STRUDELS AND PIES

A pie filled with fruit such as apples, berries, or pears will provide plenty of fiber; a graham cracker crust will add even more. Or try a crustless version such as a crisp to cut down on fat and calories.

Apple Strudel
Oodles of apple strudel without the guilt trip! Isn't that ap-peeling?

6 large baking apples, peeled, cored, and sliced (about 6 cups sliced)

2 tsp cinnamon

3–4 tbsp brown sugar (to taste)

1 tbsp lemon juice

3 tbsp whole-wheat flour

2 egg whites

½ of an egg yolk

8 sheets phyllo dough

⅓ cup graham cracker or bread crumbs

2 tsp sugar

1. Combine apples, cinnamon, brown sugar, lemon juice, and flour in a bowl. Mix well. In another bowl, blend egg whites and yolk. Preheat oven to 375°F. Spray a foil-lined baking sheet with nonstick spray. Place a sheet of phyllo dough on a dry work surface. Brush lightly with egg mixture; sprinkle lightly with crumbs. Repeat until you have 4 layers of dough. Spoon half of the filling along one long edge of dough, leaving a 1-½-inch border at bottom and sides. Fold sides inward and roll up dough. Place seam-side down on baking sheet. Repeat with remaining dough and filling. Brush tops and sides of strudel with egg mixture; sprinkle with sugar.

2. Bake at 375°F about 30 minutes, or until golden. Fruit should be tender when strudel is pierced with a knife. Best served warm. (To reheat, bake uncovered at 350°F for 15 minutes.)

Yield: 12 servings. If frozen, the dough will not be as crisp.

120 calories per serving, 1.7 g fat (0.3 g saturated), 9 mg cholesterol, 2 g protein, 25 g carbohydrate, 103 mg sodium, 111 mg potassium, 1 mg iron, 3 g fiber, 15 mg calcium

Variations

- **Blueberry-Apple Strudel:** Follow recipe for Apple Strudel (page 326), but use 3 apples and add 2 cups of blueberries. (If using frozen blueberries, thaw and drain them.) Increase brown sugar to ⅓ cup. One serving contains 124 calories, 1.6 g fat, and 26 g carbohydrate.
- **Peachy-Blueberry Strudel:** Follow recipe for Apple Strudel (page 326), but use 3 cups of peeled, sliced peaches and 2 cups of blueberries. Use ¼ cup sugar. One serving contains 117 calories, 1.5 g fat, and 24 g carbohydrate. (Nectarines can be substituted for peaches.)

Blueberry Apple Phyllo Pie

This is fabulous and so easy! What a lovely, lighter alternative to fat-laden pie.

2 cups fresh blueberries (or frozen blueberries, thawed and drained)

3 large baking apples, peeled, cored, and sliced

3 tbsp whole-wheat flour

⅓ cup brown or granulated sugar

1 tsp cinnamon

1 tbsp lemon juice

2 egg whites

½ of an egg yolk

5 sheets phyllo dough

¼ cup graham cracker or bread crumbs

1 tsp sugar

1. Preheat oven to 375°F. In a bowl, combine berries, apples, flour, sugar, cinnamon, and lemon juice. In another bowl, blend egg whites with yolk. Spray a 10-inch quiche dish with nonstick spray. Place a sheet of phyllo dough in dish, letting ends of dough hang over sides. Brush with egg; sprinkle with crumbs. Repeat until you have 4 layers of dough. Overlap each one slightly like the petals of a flower. Ends of pastry will hang over sides of pan. Reserve the last sheet of dough.

2. Spoon filling into pastry. Fold edges of pastry inwards to cover filling completely. Top with last sheet of phyllo dough, tucking ends of dough between dish and edge of pie. Brush top of pie with egg; sprinkle with sugar. Cut several slits in top of pie so steam can escape. Bake at 375°F about 45 minutes, until golden. Fruit should be tender when pie is pierced with a sharp knife. Serve warm. If desired, sprinkle with a light dusting of icing sugar.

Yield: 8 to 10 servings. If frozen, dough will not be as crisp.

156 calories per serving, 1.8 g fat (0.4 g saturated), 13 mg cholesterol, 3 g protein, 34 g carbohydrate, 115 mg sodium, 155 mg potassium, 1 mg iron, 3 g fiber, 21 mg calcium

Blueberry Crumble

Your guests won't mumble—they'll scream for more of this crispy crumble! It's terrific topped with frozen yogurt or ice cream.

Filling:
4 cups fresh or frozen blueberries (no need to thaw)
⅓ cup granulated sugar or granular Splenda
⅓ cup water
2 tbsp cornstarch
2 tbsp orange juice (preferably fresh), or cranberry or pomegranate juice

Topping:
½ cup whole-wheat flour
½ cup rolled oats (preferably large flake)
⅓ cup lightly packed brown sugar or granular Splenda
3 tbsp canola oil
½ tsp ground cinnamon

1. Preheat the oven to 350°F. Spray a 10-inch ceramic or glass pie plate with cooking spray.
2. *Filling:* Combine the blueberries, sugar, and water in a medium saucepan. Bring to a boil. Reduce heat and simmer for 5 minutes, stirring occasionally. In a small bowl, dissolve the cornstarch in the juice; stir into the blueberry mixture. Cook for 1 to 2 minutes longer or until the filling is thick and glossy. Pour into the sprayed pie plate.
3. *Topping:* Combine the flour, oats, sugar, oil, and cinnamon in a large bowl and mix together until crumbly. Sprinkle evenly over the hot blueberry mixture.
4. Bake for 30 minutes or until golden. Serve warm or at room temperature.

Yield: 10 servings. Keeps for up to 2 to 3 days in the refrigerator; reheats well. Freezes well for up to 3 months.

154 calories per serving, 28.5 g carbohydrate, 2.6 g fiber, 2 g protein, 4.8 g fat (0.4 g saturated), 0 mg cholesterol, 1 mg sodium, 90 mg potassium, 1 mg iron, 9 mg calcium. Sweet Choice—If you're using Splenda instead of sugar, one serving contains 120 calories and 18.9 g carbohydrate, making this an excellent diabetic choice.

Variations

- Instead of blueberries, substitute 4 cups of frozen mixed berries. Sliced peaches, nectarines, pears, or apples can replace part of the berries.
- *Go Nuts!* Add ½ cup slivered almonds to the topping mixture.

■ CAKES

Boost the fiber and cut the fat in your favorite cake recipes by substituting Prune Purée (page 56) for half the fat. One cup contains 12 grams of fiber!

Apple-licious Cake

This is a higher-fiber, lower-carb version of the fabulous low-fat apple cake that appears in my cookbook *Healthy Helpings* originally published as *MealLeaniYumm!* Ground almonds replace part of the flour, making it a smarter choice for those on a low GI diet. Although the fat content is slightly higher, it contains healthy monounsaturated fats from the almonds and canola oil. An apple a day will keep the doctor a-weigh!

Filling:
5 to 6 large apples, peeled, cored, and thinly sliced
3 to 4 tbsp brown sugar or granular Splenda
2 tsp ground cinnamon

Batter:
½ cup whole blanched almonds
1 large egg plus 2 egg whites (or 2 large eggs)
¾ cup granulated sugar
1 tsp pure vanilla extract
¼ cup canola oil
½ cup unsweetened applesauce
1-¼ cups whole-wheat flour
2 tsp baking powder
½ tsp ground cinnamon

1. Preheat the oven to 350°F. Spray a 7- by 11-inch glass baking dish with cooking spray.
2. In a large bowl, combine the apples with the brown sugar and cinnamon. Mix well and set aside.
3. In a food processor fitted with the steel blade, process the whole almonds until finely ground, about 25 to 30 seconds. Transfer the ground almonds to a bowl and set aside.
4. Add the egg, egg whites, sugar, vanilla extract, oil, and applesauce to the food processor; process for 2 minutes or until smooth and creamy. Don't insert the pusher into the feed tube while processing. Add the reserved ground almonds along with the flour, baking powder, and cinnamon; process just until combined.
5. Spread half the batter into the prepared pan. Spread the apple filling evenly over the batter. Top with the remaining batter and spread evenly. Some of the apples will peek through, but that's okay! Bake for 45 to 55 minutes or until the top is golden brown.

Yield: 12 servings. If frozen, the cake will become very moist. If you reheat it uncovered in a preheated 350°F oven for 10 minutes, it will taste just-baked!

238 calories per serving, 39.0 g carbohydrate, 4.7 g fiber, 4 g protein, 8.6 g fat (0.8 g saturated), 18 mg cholesterol, 101 mg sodium, 220 mg potassium, 1 mg iron, 79 mg calcium

Nutrition Notes

- *Nut Alert!* If you have nut allergies, replace the almonds with either ½ cup wheat germ or all-purpose flour.
- *Spicy News:* Recent studies have shown that as little as ¼ tsp ground cinnamon daily may improve blood glucose control. Spice up your life with cinnamon with this sinless cake!
- *GI Go!* The increased soluble fiber content of this cake comes from the addition of apples and applesauce. Increasing the soluble fiber helps to reduce the GI of baked goods. Replacing part of the flour with ground almonds helps to lower the carbohydrate content.

Apricot Prune Loaves

Prunes are being marketed as dried plums so they will seem more elegant. No matter what they're called, you'll go plum-crazy when you taste this recipe. It came from my late friend Bev Gordon, who loved to make mini loaves to give as hostess gifts. I've modified her recipe to lower the fat and sugar. These luscious loaves are sure to become a regular at your house.

Topping:
1 tbsp soft tub margarine or canola oil
¼ cup lightly packed brown sugar
⅓ cup pecans or walnuts
1 tsp ground cinnamon

Batter:
1 large egg
¼ cup canola oil
¼ cup unsweetened applesauce
1-¼ cups lightly packed brown sugar
2 tsp pure vanilla extract
1-½ cups whole-wheat flour
1 cup all-purpose flour
1 tbsp baking powder

¾ tsp baking soda

1 tsp ground cinnamon

⅛ tsp salt

1 cup buttermilk (or 1 tbsp lemon juice plus skim or soymilk to equal
1 cup)

¾ cup dried apricots

¾ cup pitted prunes

1. Preheat the oven to 350°F. Spray two 9-by 5-inch loaf pans with cooking spray.
2. In a food processor fitted with the steel blade, process the topping ingredients for 6 to 8 seconds or until crumbly. Transfer to a small bowl and reserve.
3. Process the egg, oil, applesauce, brown sugar, and vanilla for 2 minutes or until light in color. Add the flours, baking powder, baking soda, cinnamon, salt, and buttermilk; process with 6 to 8 quick on/off pulses, just until combined. Add the apricots and prunes and process with several more on/off pulses or until coarsely chopped. Pour the batter into the prepared loaf pans and spread evenly. Sprinkle with the reserved topping.
4. Bake for 45 to 55 minutes. The loaves should spring back when lightly pressed. Cool for 10 to 15 minutes before removing from the pans.

Yield: 2 loaves (20 to 24 slices). Freezes well for up to 3 months.

178 calories per slice, 30.5 g carbohydrate, 2.2 g fiber, 3 g protein, 5.4 g fat (0.6 g saturated), 11 mg cholesterol, 147 mg sodium, 215 mg potassium, 1 mg iron, 87 mg calcium

Variations

- *Mini Loaves:* Pour the batter into 4 disposable loaf pans (5-¾ by 3-¼-inches) sprayed with cooking spray. Bake for about 35 to 40 minutes. Don't remove the loaves from the pans. When cool, wrap the loaves in cellophane and tie with a ribbon. Great for gifts!
- **Apricot Prune Muffins:** Bake in sprayed muffin pans at 375°F for 20 to 25 minutes.

- **Apricot Prune Cake:** Not enough loaf pans? Spread the batter in a sprayed 9- by 13-inch or 12-cup fluted baking pan and sprinkle with topping. Bake at 350°F for 45 to 55 minutes.

Banana Cake

3 large, very ripe bananas
¼ cup canola oil
1 cup sugar
1 egg plus 2 egg whites (or 2 eggs)
1 tsp vanilla
¾ cup nonfat yogurt
1 tsp baking soda
1 tsp baking powder
1 cup whole-wheat flour
1 cup all-purpose flour

1. Preheat oven to 325°F. Spray a 7- by 11-inch Pyrex baking dish with nonstick spray. Purée bananas in the processor until smooth. Measure 1-⅓ cups purée. Beat oil, sugar, egg, egg whites, and vanilla until light, about 3 or 4 minutes. Blend in bananas. Add yogurt and process for 5 seconds. Add baking soda, baking powder, and flour. Process with quick on/off turns, until flour disappears. Spread batter evenly in prepared pan. Bake at 325°F for 45 to 55 minutes, until golden brown. Insert a cake tester into the center of cake. No batter should cling to it when done.

Yield: 15 servings. Freezes well.

177 calories per serving, 4.3 g fat (0.5 g saturated), 14 mg cholesterol, 4 g protein, 32 g carbohydrate, 128 mg sodium, 181 mg potassium, <1 mg iron, 2 g fiber, 32 mg calcium

Chef's Secret

- When you have lots of ripe bananas, purée them in the processor or mash with a potato masher. Measure 1-⅓ cups purée into each container and freeze. Freezing makes bananas taste sweeter.

Bran-ana Sour Cream Loaf

This loaf is low-fat and fiber-full. I modified my original recipe by replacing half the sugar with Splenda, substituting light sour cream for some of the bananas, and increasing the amount of whole-wheat flour. Everyone loves it!

1 large egg plus 2 egg whites (or 2 large eggs)
½ cup granulated sugar
½ cup granular Splenda
2 tbsp canola oil
1 tbsp molasses
1 tsp pure vanilla extract
1 cup All-Bran cereal
2 very ripe medium bananas (about 1 cup mashed)
½ cup light sour cream
2 tbsp lemon juice (preferably fresh)
1 cup whole-wheat flour
½ cup all-purpose flour
⅛ tsp salt
2 tsp baking powder
½ tsp baking soda

1. Preheat the oven to 350°F. Spray a 9- by 5-inch loaf pan with cooking spray.
2. In a food processor fitted with the steel blade (or in a large bowl and using an electric mixer), process (or beat) the egg, egg whites, sugar, Splenda, oil, molasses, and vanilla until light in color, about 1 minute. Add the bran cereal and process to mix well. Add the bananas, sour

cream, and lemon juice and process just until smooth. Add the flours, salt, baking powder, and baking soda; mix just until blended. Don't overprocess or the loaf will be tough.

3. Pour the batter into the prepared pan and spread evenly. Bake for 50 to 55 minutes or until golden brown. A cake tester or toothpick, when inserted in the middle, should come out clean.

Yield: 1 loaf (12 slices). Freezes well for up to 3 months.

169 calories per slice, 31 g carbohydrate, 3.3 g fiber, 5 g protein, 4.1 g fat (0.9 g saturated), 21 mg cholesterol, 194 mg sodium, 231 mg potassium, 2 mg iron, 96 mg calcium. Sweet Choice—If you replace Splenda with sugar, one slice contains 197 calories and 38.3 g carbohydrate and one muffin contains 158 calories and 30.7 g carbohydrate.

Variation

- **Bran-ana Sour Cream Muffins:** Scoop the batter into sprayed muffin pans, filling each compartment three-quarters full. You will have enough batter for about 15 muffins. Bake at 375°F for about 20 to 25 minutes. (Fill any empty compartments of muffin pans three-quarters full with water to prevent discoloration during baking.) One muffin contains 135 calories, 24.8 g carbs, 2.7 g fiber, and 3.3 g fat (0.7 g saturated).

Guilt-Free Pareve Chocolate Cake

A deep, dark secret from a light kitchen! This is a low-fat version of the pareve chocolate cake that's a family favorite from my cookbook *The Food Processor Bible*. I reduced the fat from 1-¼ cups to just ¼ cup. If you don't divulge the secret ingredient, I won't!

2⁄3 cup cocoa
2-¼ cups flour
2 cups sugar
1-½ tsp baking powder

1-½ tsp baking soda

¼ tsp salt

¾ cup coffee

¾ cup orange juice

2 eggs plus 2 egg whites (or 3 eggs)

¾ cup unsweetened applesauce or Prune Purée (page 56)

¼ cup canola oil

1. Preheat oven to 350°F. Combine all dry ingredients in the processor bowl. Process until blended, about 10 seconds. Add coffee, orange juice, eggs, egg whites, and applesauce. Start processor and add oil through the feed tube while the machine is running. Process batter for 45 seconds. Do not insert pusher in feed tube and do not overprocess.

2. Pour batter into a sprayed 12-cup Bundt pan. Bake at 350°F for 55 to 60 minutes, until cake tests done. Cool for 20 minutes before removing cake from pan.

Yield: 18 servings. Freezes well.

222 calories per serving, 4.7 g fat (0.8 g saturated), 27 mg cholesterol, 4 g protein, 43 g carbohydrate, 314 mg sodium, 125 mg potassium, 2 mg iron, 2 g fiber, 89 mg calcium

Variations

- If you don't have brewed coffee on hand, use 1-½ tsp instant coffee granules and 1-½ cups orange juice or water.
- *Skinnier Version:* If you use 1 egg and 4 egg whites, one serving will contain 219 calories, 4.4 g fat, and 13 mg cholesterol.

Light Cream Cheese Frosting

½ cup (4 oz/125 g) light cream cheese
2-½ cups icing sugar
2–3 tsp lemon juice (preferably fresh)
½ tsp grated lemon zest, optional

1.   Combine all ingredients in the processor and blend until smooth.

60 calories per serving (¹⁄₂₄th of a recipe), 0.9 g fat (0.6 g saturated), 3 mg cholesterol, <1 g protein, 13 g carbohydrate, 15 mg sodium, 9 mg potassium, trace iron, 0 g fiber, 6 mg calcium

Moist 'n' Luscious Carrot Cake

Dave Horan's favorite! You won't believe it's low-fat. Most low-fat carrot cakes include buttermilk or yogurt, but I was determined to create a dairy-free cake. My testers loved the results. If you must have icing on your cake, use Light Cream Cheese Frosting (see recipe above). Guiltless pleasure!

3 cups grated carrots (6–8 carrots)
1 egg plus 2 egg whites (or 2 eggs)
3 tbsp canola oil
1-¾ cups sugar
2 tsp vanilla
¾ cup unsweetened applesauce
2-½ cups flour (I use half whole-wheat flour)
1-½ tsp baking powder
1-½ tsp baking soda
1 tbsp cinnamon
¼ tsp salt
2 tbsp wheat germ
½ cup raisins or mini chocolate chips
Light Cream Cheese Frosting, if desired

1. Preheat oven to 350°F. Spray a 9- by 13-inch baking pan with nonstick spray. Grate carrots, measure 3 cups and set aside. Beat egg, egg whites, oil, sugar, vanilla, and applesauce. Beat until light, about 2 to 3 minutes. Add grated carrots and mix well. Combine flour, baking powder, baking soda, cinnamon, salt, and wheat germ. Add to batter and mix just until flour disappears. Stir in raisins or chocolate chips. Pour batter into prepared pan. Bake at 350°F for 45 to 50 minutes, or until a toothpick inserted into the center of the cake comes out with no batter clinging to it.

Yield: 24 servings. Freezes well.

144 calories per serving (without frosting), 2.2 g fat (0.2 g saturated), 9 mg cholesterol, 3 g protein, 30 g carbohydrate, 135 mg sodium, 130 mg potassium, <1 mg iron, 2 g fiber, 14 mg calcium

Zucchini Cake with Almonds and Raisins

This large, moist cake contains whole-wheat flour, vegetables, fruit, and nuts, with half the sugar of a traditional zucchini cake. Zucchini is a terrific source of lutein, which helps prevent macular degeneration. You'll see how quickly this cake disappears.

1 cup all-purpose flour
1 cup plus 2 tbsp whole-wheat flour
2 tsp baking powder
1 tsp baking soda
⅛ tsp salt
1 tbsp ground cinnamon
1 unpeeled medium zucchini, ends trimmed (about 2 cups grated)
2 large eggs plus 2 egg whites (or 3 large eggs)
1 cup lightly packed brown sugar
½ cup canola oil
½ cup unsweetened applesauce
2 tsp pure vanilla extract

2 tbsp lemon or orange juice (preferably fresh)
½ cup slivered almonds
½ cup raisins

1. Preheat the oven to 350°F. Spray a 12-cup fluted tube pan with cooking spray.
2. In a food processor fitted with the steel blade, process the flours, baking powder, baking soda, salt, and cinnamon for 10 seconds or until blended. Transfer to a bowl.
3. Grate the zucchini; you should end up with about 2 cups, loosely packed.
4. In the food processor, process the eggs, brown sugar, oil, applesauce, and vanilla extract for 2 minutes or until smooth and creamy. Don't insert the pusher into the feed tube while processing. Add the grated zucchini and lemon juice; process 10 seconds longer. Add the reserved dry ingredients; process with several quick on/off pulses, just until blended. Add the almonds and raisins; process with 2 or 3 quick on/off pulses to combine. Pour the batter into the prepared tube pan and spread evenly.
5. Bake for 50 to 60 minutes or until a cake tester or toothpick inserted into the center comes out clean. Cool the cake in the pan for 15 minutes before inverting onto a cake plate and removing it from the pan.

Yield: 18 servings. Freezes well for up to 3 months.

200 calories per serving, 28.4 g carbohydrate, 2.1 g fiber, 4 g protein, 8.6 g fat (0.8 g saturated), 24 mg cholesterol, 162 mg sodium, 192 mg potassium, 1 mg iron, 64 mg calcium

Variation

- Substitute walnuts for almonds and dried cranberries or semi-sweet chocolate chips for raisins.

Chef's Secrets

- *Company's Coming!* Sift 2 tbsp icing sugar on top of the cooled cake. Alternatively, prepare a cream cheese frosting, adding a little extra lemon juice until it reaches the consistency of a glaze. Drizzle the glaze over the cooled cake—your guests will go "glazy" over it!

SNACKS

WHAT'S INSIDE

Plenty of high fiber snacks are available in the supermarket; buy them pre-packaged and carry with you in case of the munchies. The following are good fiber-rich options:

- whole-wheat pretzels (try health food stores)
- dried fruit and vegetables
- nuts

Other quick snacks that are full of fiber include raw, precut vegetables such as baby carrots, celery or bell peppers, broccoli, and cauliflower. Grocery stores sell them as snacks or as a mix ready for stir-fry dishes. When they're cut, cleaned, and prepackaged, they're easy to grab from the fridge. Fruit, of course, comes in its own package, and it's full of fiber.

■ DIPS AND SPREADS

A high fiber dip or spread, combined with whole-grain breads, crackers, or vegetables, can really boost your fiber intake.

Baked Tortilla Chips

Chip, chip hooray! These tasty triangles are delicious with your favorite dip, spread, or salsa.

> 6 10-inch whole-wheat flour or corn tortillas
> 2 egg whites, lightly beaten
> 6 tbsp sesame seeds
> Kosher salt
> Italian seasoning

1. Preheat the oven to 400°F. Line a baking sheet with parchment paper or foil sprayed with cooking spray.
2. Using a pastry brush or paper towel, brush each tortilla with a light coating of egg white. Sprinkle with the sesame seeds, salt, and seasoning. Evenly stack the tortillas on top of each other and, using a sharp knife,

cut into wedges (first cut the stack in half, then into quarters, then into eighths, like cutting a pizza).

3. Arrange the tortilla wedges, sesame seed-side up, in a single layer on the prepared baking sheet. Bake uncovered for 8 to 10 minutes or until the tops are crisp and golden. Watch carefully to prevent burning.

Yield: 12 servings (48 triangles). Keeps 2 to 3 weeks at room temperature in a re-sealable plastic bag. If freezing, pack and store carefully in a freezer container as they are fragile. These freeze for 2 to 3 months.

65 calories per serving (4 triangles), 10.7 g carbohydrate, 1.4 g fiber, 4 g protein, 2.3 g fat (0 g saturated), 0 mg cholesterol, 103 mg sodium, 50 mg potassium, 1 mg iron, 20 mg calcium

Variations

- **Pita Chips:** Use pita bread instead of tortillas. Split each pita into two rounds and prepare as directed.
- Instead of egg white, brush each tortilla lightly with extra virgin olive oil and sprinkle with minced garlic. Add a sprinkling of dried basil, thyme, oregano, rosemary, or a barbecue seasoning mixture.
- Sprinkle with Parmesan cheese or sesame seeds, if desired.

Nutrition Notes

- The nutritional analysis was done using whole-wheat flour tortillas, which have a GI value of 30. Corn tortillas (GI value 52) are an excellent alternative for those who are gluten-intolerant.
- Tortillas come in different sizes and contain different amounts of fat, calories, and fiber, so check the nutrient label when shopping and compare different brands.
- Don't use low-carb tortillas to make these chips—they'll have a cardboard-like texture. Low-carb tortillas taste best in their original soft state, so use them for wraps, or cut them in wedges and serve them lightly toasted with dips. One low-carb tortilla contains about 12 g of carbohydrates and 9 g of fiber.

Basic Skinny Dip
(See recipe, page 110)

Black Bean Dip
(See recipe, page 110)

Chickpea Mock Chopped Liver
Canned lentils can be substituted for chickpeas.

  3 medium onions
  1-½ cups cooked or canned chickpeas, rinsed and drained
  2 tbsp almonds or walnuts, optional
  2 hard-boiled eggs (or 1 hard-boiled egg plus 2 hard-boiled whites)
  Salt and pepper, to taste
  1 tsp honey

1. Preheat oven to 400°F. Place unpeeled onions on a baking sheet and bake for 40 minutes, until soft. (Or pierce onions in 3 or 4 places with a sharp knife; place on a plate and microwave on HIGH for 6 to 8 minutes.) Cool slightly; remove peel. Combine all ingredients in processor. Process 30 seconds, until finely chopped. If mixture seems dry, blend in a little water. Chill before serving.

Yield: About 2-¾ cups. Mixture keeps for 3 or 4 days in the refrigerator. It can be frozen, but season mixture lightly because the pepper's flavor will become stronger.

74 calories per ¼ cup, 2.4 g fat (0.4 g saturated), 39 mg cholesterol, 4 g protein, 10 g carbohydrate, 14 mg sodium, 132 mg potassium, <1 mg iron, 2 g fiber, 25 mg calcium

Easy Spinach Dip

An enlightened version of an old favorite. This dip is usually served in a hollowed-out round pumpernickel or country bread.

> 10 oz pkg (300 g) frozen chopped spinach, thawed and squeezed dry
> 1 can (8 oz/227 ml) water chestnuts, drained and chopped
> 4 green onions, chopped
> ½ pkg dehydrated vegetable soup mix
> 1-½ cups nonfat yogurt
> ½ cup fat-free or light mayonnaise

1. Combine all ingredients and mix well. Serve chilled with assorted crudités and cubes of bread.

Yield: About 3-½ cups. Dip keeps about 3 or 4 days in the refrigerator.

7 calories per tbsp, 0.1 g fat (0 g saturated), trace cholesterol, <1 g protein, 1 g carbohydrate, 25 mg sodium, 33 mg potassium, trace iron, trace fiber, 16 mg calcium

Ethel Cherry's Smoky Eggplant Dip

(See recipe, page 112)

Garden Vegetable Hummus

(See recipe, page 113)

Green Pea Guacamole

With this recipe, you won't have to worry about finding ripe avocados. Frozen green peas will be ready when you are, and they won't turn brown when mashed. One cup of green peas contains 111 calories and only half a gram of fat!

1 cup frozen green peas
1 clove garlic
2–3 tsp fresh lime juice (to taste)
3 tbsp mild or medium salsa
3 tbsp nonfat yogurt or sour cream
½ tsp extra virgin olive oil, optional
Salt and pepper, optional
Pinch of cumin

1. Microwave peas on HIGH for 2 minutes, just until defrosted. In the food processor, drop garlic through the feed tube and process until minced. Add lime juice and peas. Process until minced, about 1 minute, scraping down sides of bowl several times. Blend in salsa, yogurt, and oil, if using. Season to taste. Transfer mixture to a bowl, cover and refrigerate until ready to serve. (Can be made up to one day in advance.)

Yield: about 1 cup. Do not freeze. Delicious as a dip with Pita or Baked Tortilla Chips (page 342).

9 calories per tbsp, 0 g fat (0 g saturated), 0 mg cholesterol, <1 g protein, 2 g carbohydrate, 19 mg sodium, 27 mg potassium, trace iron, <1 g fiber, 9 mg calcium

Guacamole with Hearts of Palm

The inspiration for this Venezuelan variation of guacamole, known as *guasacaca*, comes from my friend Elena Eder of Miami. Elena adds hearts of palm to reduce the calories and fat. It's traditionally served with grilled meats or fish, tortillas, pita bread, or flatbread.

> 1 can (14 oz/398 ml) hearts of palm, well-drained
> 2 tbsp fresh cilantro and/or parsley
> 1 small onion
> 1 clove garlic (about 1 tsp minced)
> ½ red pepper, cut in chunks
> 1 medium tomato, cored and quartered
> 1 medium avocado, peeled and pitted
> 1 tbsp extra virgin olive oil
> 1 tbsp lemon juice (preferably fresh)
> ½ tsp salt
> Freshly ground black pepper
> ¼ tsp cayenne pepper or chili powder

1. In a food processor fitted with the steel blade, process the hearts of palm and cilantro, using quick on/off pulses, until finely chopped. Transfer to a medium mixing bowl—you should have about 1 cup.
2. Process the onion, garlic, and red pepper with quick on/off pulses, until coarsely chopped. Add the tomato, avocado, oil, lemon juice, salt, pepper, and cayenne. Continue processing with several quick on/off pulses, until the vegetables are coarsely chopped. Add to the hearts of palm and mix well. Adjust seasonings to taste.

Yield: About 3 cups. Keeps 4 to 5 days, in a tightly sealed container, in the refrigerator. Don't freeze.

46 calories per ¼ cup serving, 3.2 g carbohydrate, 1.6 g fiber, 1 g protein, 3.7 g fat (0.5 g saturated), 0 mg cholesterol, 127 mg sodium, 140 mg potassium, 0 mg iron, 9 mg calcium

Chef's Secrets

- *Go for Green!* You don't have to worry about the avocado turning brown in this recipe—the addition of hearts of palm solves the problem.
- *Hot, Hot, Hot!* This traditional South American dish is made with red and green chili peppers, but I used red pepper and kicked up the heat with cayenne.

Healthier Hummus

(See recipe, page 114)

Luscious Lentil Paté

(See recipe, page 116)

Molly Naimer's Green Pea Mock Liver

Molly Naimer lived at Manoir Montefiore, a Montreal senior residence where I was the food consultant. If you make her recipe, perhaps you'll also live into your 90s! When I asked Molly if this dish could be frozen, she replied, "I don't know. I never had leftovers. It was always eaten up!"

1 large onion, finely diced
1 tbsp canola oil (approximately)
19 oz (540 ml) can green peas, drained and mashed
4 hard-boiled eggs, peeled and grated
8 walnut halves, chopped (not ground!)
Salt and pepper, to taste

1. In a nonstick skillet, brown onion in oil until crispy. Combine with remaining ingredients and mix well. Season to taste. Refrigerate to blend flavors. Use as a vegetarian alternative to chopped liver.

Yield: about 3 cups. Mixture keeps for 3 or 4 days in the fridge.

71 calories per ¼ cup, 4 g fat (0.7 g saturated), 73 mg cholesterol, 4 g protein, 5 g carbohydrate, 95 mg sodium, 98 mg potassium, <1 mg iron, 1 g fiber, 18 mg calcium

Chef's Secrets

- If you discard 2 of the yolks, ¼ cup of the above spread will contain 64 calories, 38 mg cholesterol and 3.2 g fat (0.5 g saturated).
- *Compare the Difference!* An equal amount of chopped chicken livers with egg and onion has 132 calories, 212 mg cholesterol, and 10.4 g fat (3.2 g saturated).

Pumpkin Hummus
(See recipe, page 119)

Roasted Eggplant Spread
(See recipe, page 120)

White Bean Dip
(See recipe, page 130)

■ MISCELLANEOUS

Crunchy Roasted Chickpeas (Nahit)

This addictive snack comes from two "foodie" friends. Caryn Bloomberg of Columbus, Ohio, loves them because they satisfy her cravings when she has the munchies. Omi Cantor of Framingham, Massachusetts, remembers these being served at her synagogue after services. Crunch away!

> 1 can (19 oz/540 ml) chickpeas or 2 cups cooked chickpeas
> Salt, pepper, and garlic powder
> Sweet or smoked paprika

1. Preheat the oven to 350°F. Line a rimmed baking sheet with foil and spray with cooking spray.
2. If using canned chickpeas, drain, rinse, and pat dry with paper towels. Combine the chickpeas with salt, pepper, garlic powder, and paprika in a medium bowl and mix well.
3. Spread in a single layer on the prepared baking sheet. Roast, uncovered, for 50 to 60 minutes or until crisp and golden, stirring them every 15 minutes.
4. Remove from the oven and let cool. Store at room temperature in a loosely covered bowl or container. Serve at room temperature.

Yield: About 1-¼ cups (5 servings of ¼ cup each). We don't know how long they keep because they never last long enough! Don't freeze.

114 calories per serving, 21.7 g carbohydrate, 4.2 g fiber, 5 g protein, 1.1 g fat (0.1 saturated), 0 mg cholesterol, 287 mg sodium, 165 mg potassium, 1 mg iron, 31 mg calcium

Cheater's Chickpeas

- Season canned, drained chickpeas with salt and lots of pepper, but don't bother roasting them. Cover and refrigerate. Enjoy them as a snack.

Chef's Secrets

- *Spice It Up!* Chili powder, cumin, and/or curry powder add a spicy kick to these crunchy nibbles. Or use your favorite mixture of herbs and spices. Always different, always delicious!
- *Soy Good!* Omit the seasonings and lightly drizzle the chickpeas with tamari or soy sauce, then roast as directed.
- *Easy-Peasy!* Sprinkle on top of salads instead of nuts.

Edamame

Edamame (pronounced eh-dah-MAH-meh) means "beans on branches." It is the Japanese name for soybeans still in their pods. Available fresh or frozen, edamame makes a healthy snack or appetizer and is delicious in salads and stir-fries. Al Jolson would probably have branched out his repertoire and sung about these for his Mammy if he had tasted them.

1 lb (454 g) frozen, unshelled edamame
2 cloves garlic (peeling isn't necessary)
Kosher or sea salt

1. In a large pot, bring 4 quarts of salted water to a boil on high heat. Add edamame and garlic. Bring water back to a boil, then cook uncovered for about 6 to 8 minutes or until tender-crisp. Do not overcook or they will become mushy.
2. Drain well but don't rinse. Discard the garlic. Spread the edamame out on a baking sheet lined with paper towels and let cool.
3. Transfer to a platter or bowl and sprinkle with Kosher salt. Serve at room temperature.

Yield: 6 servings. Don't freeze.

133 calories per 100 g (edible portion), 12 g carbohydrate, 5.3 g fiber, 11 g protein, 4.0 g fat (0 g saturated), 0 mg cholesterol, 40 mg sodium, potassium (unavailable), 2 mg iron, 67 mg calcium

Chef's Secrets
- *Pod-cast the News!* Pull the pods through your teeth to extract the soybeans, or squeeze the beans directly from the pods into your mouth with your fingers. Don't eat the pods. (Have an extra bowl for the discarded pods.)
- *Fresh vs. Frozen!* Fresh edamame takes longer to cook than frozen. Cook fresh edamame, in the pod, in salted water for 20 minutes or until tender. (If frozen, edamame takes 6 to 8 minutes to cook.) Drain well, but don't rinse. The salt will cling to the outside of the pods.

Nutrition Note
- Edamame resembles sugar snap peas and are very easy to digest. This bright green vegetable is very high in protein and fiber. One half cup of edamame contains 8 grams of soy protein, which helps reduce cholesterol. Oy, soy healthy!

Tomato Tidbits

Good things come in small packages. These tasty tidbits are very versatile. Enjoy them as a snack, add them to a vegetable tray, or use them in salads, pasta, or grains. Nibble a-weigh!

> 2 containers (about 4 cups) grape or cherry tomatoes
> 2 tsp extra virgin olive oil
> Salt, freshly ground black pepper, and dried basil

1. Preheat the oven to 250°F. Line a baking sheet with foil and spray with cooking spray.
2. Cut the tomatoes in half and place, cut-side up, in a single layer on the baking sheet. Drizzle with oil and season with salt, pepper, and basil to taste. Bake, uncovered, for 2 to 3 hours or until the tomato halves are shriveled and somewhat chewy. Don't bother turning them over. Cooking time will vary depending on the size and moisture content of tomatoes.

3.   Remove from the oven and cool completely before serving.

Yield: About 2 cups (8 servings of ¼ cup each). Recipe doubles easily. These keep in the refrigerator for several weeks (but they're so good, they never last that long). Freezes well for up to 2 months.

23 calories per serving, 2.9 g carbohydrate, 0.9 g fiber, 1 g protein, 1.3 g fat (0.2 g saturated), 0 mg cholesterol, 4 mg sodium, 177 mg potassium, 0 mg iron, 8 mg calcium

Chef's Secret

- *Chewy or Crispy?* If you prefer them chewier, store in a tightly covered container in the refrigerator. If you prefer them more crispy, keep them uncovered at room temperature. The choice is yours.

■ SWEET STUFF

Fortunately, a high fiber diet doesn't preclude sweets!

Anytime Breakfast Cookies
(See recipe, page 28)

Apple Turnovers
If you are not concerned with the fat content, brush each sheet of phyllo dough very lightly with canola oil instead of the egg mixture.

6 large apples, peeled, cored, and sliced
2 tsp cinnamon
3–4 tbsp brown sugar
1 tbsp lemon juice
2 egg whites
½ of an egg yolk
8 sheets phyllo dough
3 tbsp graham cracker or bread crumbs

1. Cook apples, cinnamon, and brown sugar in a saucepan until soft, about 6 to 8 minutes. Stir in lemon juice. In a small bowl, blend egg whites with yolk. Preheat oven to 400°F. Spray a foil-lined baking sheet with nonstick spray. Place a sheet of phyllo on a dry work surface. Brush lightly with egg. Top with another sheet of dough; sprinkle lightly with crumbs. Cut into 3 long strips.
2. Place a spoonful of drained apple filling 1 inch from the bottom of each strip. Fold dough upwards to cover filling. Then fold right bottom corner of dough upward diagonally to meet left edge, making a triangle. Continue folding from side to side until folded. Repeat with remaining dough and filling. Place triangles seam-side down on baking sheet. Brush lightly with egg mixture. Bake at 400°F for 18 to 20 minutes, until golden. (To reheat, bake uncovered at 350°F for 10 minutes.)

Yield: 12 servings. If frozen, the dough will not be as crisp.

105 calories per serving, 1.5 g fat (0.3 g saturated), 9 mg cholesterol, 2 g protein, 22 g carbohydrate, 94 mg sodium, 101 mg potassium, <1 mg iron, 3 g fiber, 14 mg calcium

Chunky Monkey
(See recipe page 60)

Fruit Smoothies
(See recipe page 60)

Homemade Cereal Bars
(See recipe page 30)

Mango Berry Smoothie
(See recipe page 62)

Trail Mix
Keep this tasty mix handy for a quick fix when you get a snack attack. Dividing it into small, re-sealable bags ensures portion control. Now all you need is self-control!

> 1 cup toasted mixed nuts (walnuts, almonds, pecans, peanuts, and/or soy nuts)
> ½ cup semi-sweet chocolate chips (regular or miniature)
> ¼ cup dried cranberries or raisins
> ¼ cup toasted pumpkin seeds
> 2 cups toasted oat cereal (e.g., Cheerios) or other unsweetened breakfast cereal

1. Combine the nuts, chocolate chips, cranberries or raisins, pumpkin seeds, and cereal in a medium bowl and mix well.
2. Divide into 8 small re-sealable plastic bags.

Yield: 4 cups (8 servings of ½ cup each). Store in a cool, dry place. Keeps for 1 to 2 months, but it never lasts that long. Don't freeze.

181 calories per serving, 18.1 g carbohydrate, 2.7 g fiber, 4 g protein, 12.1 g fat (2.8 g saturated), 0 mg cholesterol, 55 mg sodium, 166 mg potassium, 3 mg iron, 47 mg calcium

Variations

- *Nut Alert!* If you have concerns about nut allergies, omit them and add any of the other suggested ingredients. Use your imagination. Calorie counts will vary.
- *Kid Stuff:* Instead of chocolate chips, substitute M&M's or miniature marshmallows.
- *Tropical Fruit Mix:* Instead of cranberries or raisins, substitute slivered dried apricots, dried pineapple, or mango.
- *Crunchy Munchies!* Instead of toasted oat cereal, use bite-sized shredded wheat cereal or pretzels.
- *Hop on Pop!* Substitute popcorn for nuts and/or cereal.

CHAPTER NINE

CHILD-FRIENDLY MEALS

WHAT'S INSIDE

If you're feeding a child, you know that kids follow different rules when it comes to eating. Most are reluctant to try unfamiliar ingredients—a big problem when you're hoping to overhaul their diet.

But you can often win children over to a new food if you keep offering it. Give them a small portion of one new ingredient along with food they already like. Try giving it to them at the beginning of the meal when they're the most hungry. Don't threaten or force them to eat it, as this tactic usually backfires. Let them try it when they're ready—it may take as many as 20 times!

Another trick is to hide fiber in foods they enjoy: Serve macaroni and cheese with whole-grain pasta. Mix bran into hamburger patties. Batter chicken or fish fingers in whole-grain bread crumbs. Serve white whole-wheat bread if they're suspicious of the brown variety. There are also white breads fortified with added fiber—kids can't tell the difference.

You can also rely on the high fiber food they're already fond of—children often love baby carrots, frozen peas, corn, and fruit. In fact, fruit is probably your biggest ally in your effort to boost the fiber in your child's diet. Serve it with abandon—whole, sliced, puréed in smoothies, mixed in pancakes.

■ BREAKFAST

Cold cereals that contain goods amounts of fiber include Wheaties, Frosted Mini-Wheats, Raisin Bran and Quaker Oats. Unfortunately, as with many cold cereals, these choices contain high levels of sugar. You may be able to find lower-sugar, high fiber cereals in a health food store. Another quick, healthful breakfast includes fruit and whole-wheat toast (with the crusts removed, of course) topped with peanut butter. Or whip up a fiber-full smoothie made of milk and fruit.

Apple Blue-Peary Sauce
(See recipe, page 32)

Blueberry Cornmeal Pancakes
(See recipe, page 33)

Blueberry Corn Muffins
(See recipe, page 49)

Bran-ana Sour Cream Muffins
(See recipe, page 336)

Bran and Date Muffins
(See recipe, page 51)

Chunky Monkey
(See recipe, page 60)

Cinnamon Apple Pancakes
(See recipe, page 35)

Fabulous Fruit Crisp
(See recipe, page 63)

Fruit Smoothies
(See recipe, page 60)

Granola
(See recipe, page 29)

High Fiber Bread
(See recipe, page 42)

Homemade Cereal Bars
(See recipe, page 30)

Homemade Fruit Pancakes
(See recipe, page 36)

Homemade Whole-Wheat Bread (Processor Method)
(See recipe, page 43)

Jumbleberry Crisp
(See recipe, page 65)

Mango Berry Smoothie
(See recipe, page 62)

Oatmeal Wheat Germ Bread
(See recipe, page 45)

Peachy Crumb Crisp
(See recipe, page 67)

■ LUNCH

For school lunches, go with whole-grain bread or crackers. Kids often like Triscuits, Wheat Thins, and rice crackers made with brown rice. You can do quite well with peanut butter sandwiches on whole-wheat or fiber-enriched bread. A piece of fruit or bag of baby carrots will make it a high fiber meal indeed.

If you're serving lunch at home, try whole-wheat pita or whole-grain tortilla chips with bean dip or mild salsa. Kids like to dip!

Autumn Vegetable Soup
(See recipe, page 70)

Black Bean Dip
(See recipe, page 110)

Black Bean Soup
(See recipe, page 73)

Easy Enchiladas
(See recipe, page 156)

Hi-Fiber Vegetarian Lasagna
(See recipe, page 146)

Quick Pea Soup
(See recipe, page 80)

Rozie's Freeze with Ease Turkey Chili
(See recipe, page 142)

■ DINNER

The best time to introduce new foods is when the family is eating together. If children see parents or older children enjoying a new food, they'll often want to try it themselves.

Almost Meat Lasagna

(See recipe, page 288)

Black Bean and Corn Casserole

(See recipe, page 291)

Cheater's Hi-Fiber Pasta Sauce

(See recipe, page 270)

Chicken Fajitas

(See recipe, page 240)

Curried Carrot and Cashew Soup

(See recipe, page 176)

Glazed Sweet Potatoes

(See recipe, page 206)

Homemade Baked Beans

(See recipe, page 209)

Honey-Glazed Carrots

(See recipe, page 210)

No-Fry Almond Schnitzel
(See recipe, page 250)

Nutty-Baked Chicken
(See recipe, page 252)

Pecan-Crusted Tilapia
(See recipe, page 232)

Penne with Roasted Vegetable Purée
(See recipe, page 276)

Potato and Carrot Purée
(See recipe, page 217)

Secret Ingredient Sweet and Sour Meatballs
(See recipe, page 268)

Squish Squash Soup
(See recipe, page 183)

Squished Squash
(See recipe, page 226)

Sweet Potato "Fries"
(See recipe, page 227)

■ DESSERT

You won't need to work too hard to convince kids to try these dishes!

Apple Strudel
(See recipe, page 326)

Apple-licious Cake
(See recipe, page 330)

Apricot Prune Loaves
(See recipe, page 333)

Banana Cake
(See recipe, page 334)

Berry Fool
(See recipe, page 302)

Berry Mango Sherbet
(See recipe, page 303)

Best Oatmeal Cookies
(See recipe, page 318)

Blueberry Crumble
(See recipe, page 329)

Brownie Cookies
(See recipe, page 320)

Chocolate Chewies
(See recipe, page 321)

Chocolate Chip Cookies
(See recipe, page 322)

Frozen Peanut Butter Mousse
(See recipe, page 305)

Guilt-Free Pareve Chocolate Cake
(See recipe, page 336)

Luscious Lemon Berry Mousse
(See recipe, page 306)

Mock Banana Soft Ice Cream
(See recipe, page 307)

Moist 'n' Luscious Carrot Cake
(See recipe, page 338)

Pumpkin Cheesecake
(See recipe, page 308)

Slimmer Hello Dollies
(See recipe, page 325)

Strawberry and Banana Frozen Yogurt
(See recipe, page 310)

Strawberry Buttermilk Sherbet

(See recipe, page 311)

■ SNACKS

Can you think of a time-honored kid snack that's full of fiber? Popcorn!

Baked Tortilla Chips

(See recipe, page 342)

Trail Mix

(See recipe, page 355)

FIBER CONTENT OF SELECTED FOODS

Grains		Total Fiber (grams)
Wheat bran, dry	¼ cup	6
Barley, cooked	½ cup	4
Bulgur, cooked	½ cup	4
Brown rice, cooked	½ cup	2
Wheat germ, ready to eat	¼ cup	4
Cracked wheat, cooked	½ cup	3
Multigrain or granola bread	1 slice	2
Spaghetti, whole-wheat	1 cup	4
Spaghetti	1 cup	2
Whole-wheat bread	1 slice	2
White bread	1 slice	1
Legumes and Nuts		**Total Fiber (grams)**
Lentils, cooked	½ cup	8
Lima beans	½ cup	7
Beans, baked	½ cup	6
Kidney beans	½ cup	6
Navy beans	½ cup	6
Pigeon peas, cooked	½ cup	6
Green peas, cooked	½ cup	4
Peanuts, dry roasted	¼ cup	3
Walnuts	¼ cup	2
Filberts, raw	10 nuts	1

Fruits		Total Fiber (grams)
Pear, fresh	1 large	5
Apple, fresh	1 medium	4
Blueberries, fresh	1 cup	4
Plum, fresh	5 small	4
Strawberries, fresh	1 cup	4
Apricot, fresh	3 fruits	3
Banana, fresh	1 medium	3
Orange, fresh	1 medium	3
Apricot, dried	5 half	2
Cherries, fresh	10 fruits	2
Dates	3 fruits	2
Peach, fresh	1 medium	2
Prune, dried	3 fruits	2
Raisins	¼ cup	2
Cantaloupe	¼ medium	1
Grapefruit	½ medium	1
Grapes, fresh, without seeds	20	1
Grapes, fresh, without seeds	½ cup	1
Vegetables		**Total Fiber (grams)**
Parsnips, cooked	½ cup	4
Carrots, cooked	½ cup	3
Brussels sprouts, cooked	½ cup	3
Potato, baked with skin	1 medium	3
Spinach, cooked	½ cup	3
Winter squash, cooked	½ cup	3
Beans, string	½ cup	2
Cabbage, cooked	½ cup	2
Cauliflower, cooked	½ cup	2
Corn, cooked	½ cup	2

Vegetables, continued		Total Fiber (grams)
Sweet potato, baked	½ cup	2
Turnip, cooked	½ cup	2
Broccoli, cooked	½ cup	1
Kale, cooked	½ cup	1
Summer squash, cooked	½ cup	1
Tomato, raw	1 medium	1
Zucchini, cooked	½ cup	1
Cereals		**Total Fiber (grams)**
Fiber One	½ cup	14
All-Bran	⅔ cup	13
All-Bran with extra fiber	½ cup	13
100% Bran	½ cup	12
Bran Buds	⅓ cup	12
Raisin Bran	¾ cup	6
Bran Flakes, without raisins	¾ cup	5
Complete Bran Flakes	¾ cup	5
Wheat Chex	⅔ cup	5
Bran Chex, Multi	⅔ cup	4
Grape-Nuts Flakes	1 cup	4
Nutri-Grain Golden Wheat	¾ cup	4
Oatmeal	1 cup	4
Total	1 cup	4
Cheerios	1-¼ cup	4
Original Frosted Mini-Wheats	4 large pieces	4
Basic 4	¾ cup	3

Cereals, continued		Total Fiber (grams)
Complete Oat Bran Flakes	⅔ cup	3
Cracklin' Oat Bran	⅓ cup	3
Mueslix, Raisin, Almond, Dates	½ cup	3
Shredded Wheat	⅔ cup	3
Granola, low fat with raisins	½ cup	3
Grape-Nuts	¼ cup	2
Heartland Granola	¼ cup	2
Just Right Fruit and Nut	¾ cup	2
Smart Start	1 cup	2
Wheaties	1 cup	2
Corn Flakes	1-¼ cup	1
Smacks	¾ cup	1
Special K	1-⅓ cup	1

Amounts are rounded to the nearest whole number.

Source: Minnesota Nutrient Data Base 4.04, Tufts University School of Medicine, Boston, MA, Revised 3/02

RECICE INDEX

S

Made in the USA
Middletown, DE
30 December 2017